J.-U. Stolzenburg • Matthew T. Gettman • Evangelos N. Liatsikos (Eds.)

Endoscopic Extraperitoneal Radical Prostatectomy
Laparoscopic and Robot-Assisted Surgery

J.-U. Stolzenburg · M.T. Gettman · E.N. Liatsikos   (Eds.)

Endoscopic Extraperitoneal Radical Prostatectomy

Laparoscopic and Robot-Assisted Surgery

With 197 Figures and 10 Tables

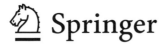
Springer

Stolzenburg, Jens-Uwe, MD, FRCS (Ed)
Professor and Chairman
Department of Urology
Head of International Training
Centre of Urologic Laparoscopy
University of Leipzig
Liebigstraße 20
04103 Leipzig, Germany
e-mail: stolj@medizin.uni-leipzig.de

Gettman, Matthew T., MD
Associate Professor
Department of Urology
Mayo Clinic
Gonda 7S, 200 1st Street SW
Rochester, MN 55905, USA
e-mail: Gettman.Matthew@mayo.edu

Liatsikos, Evangelos N., MD, PhD
Assistant Professor of Urology
Department of Urology
University of Patras, School of Medicine
26500 Rio, Patras, Greece
e-mail: Liatsikos@yahoo.com

Library of Congress Control Number: 2007934520

ISBN-978-3-540-45533-2   Springer Berlin Heidelberg New York

Springer is a part of Springer Science + Business Media
springer.com

© Springer-Verlag Berlin Heidelberg 2007

Medical Editor: Dr. Ute Heilmann, Heidelberg, Germany
Desk Editor: Dörthe Mennecke-Bühler, Heidelberg, Germany
Cover design: Frido Steinen-Broo, eStudio Calamar, Spain
Reproduction and Typesetting: am-productions GmbH, Wiesloch, Germany
Production: L$_E$-TEX Jelonek, Schmidt & Vöckler GbR, Leipzig, Germany

Printed on acid-free paper   27/3100 – YL – 5 4 3 2 1 0

Foreword

Minimally invasive interventions were a source of controversy as early as the beginning of the 1960s in stone removal. A group of young, aggressive urologists gradually shortened the standard approach to the kidney to a few centimetres, developed special instruments for this purpose, and entered into competition with the general surgeons who were carrying out cholecystectomies via mini-incisions. The arguments – shortening hospital stay, decreasing the need for postoperative pain therapy – were the same, until PNL and ESWL achieved better results.

Age and experience have always been the enemies of progress, but this did not prevent the development of laparoscopic techniques in urology, beginning with the detection of cryptorchid testes and retroperitoneal lymphadenectomy. Ten years ago I counselled one of my most dextrous pupils to avoid laparoscopy. He ignored my advice and is now one of the most sought-after urologists in Belgium.

In the evolution of surgical techniques the wheel of history has often rolled backwards. The widespread use of clamps in intestinal surgery is perhaps one of the most instructive examples of a broad return to conventional techniques, with the newer methods becoming restricted to particular indications.

It is only natural to mistrust a new technique – in this case EERPE – that one cannot perform oneself.

In the field of laparoscopy the investment in robots is so immense that a retreat in the foreseeable future seems unlikely. In the USA – the land of unlimited opportunities – robot-assisted radical prostate surgery has become one of the financial pillars of 500 urological clinics, with up to three operations per day. It thus seems likely that industry will exert more influence than ever on the diffusion of laparoscopic techniques.

Word of mouth, however, remains the strongest influence on individual patients, who gravitate to the centres where satisfaction is highest. Distance and time play an ever-decreasing role in their decisions.

The Centre of Urologic Laparoscopy at the University of Leipzig is among the leading institutions in terms of numbers of patients treated, and is peerless in the number of courses offered each year and the number of participants. This book is thus a product of 10 years' experience of performing and teaching EERPE. All that has been learned is contained between its covers.

The reader just needs to glance at the chapter on topographical anatomy to become enthralled by the innovative three-dimensional functional depiction of the pelvic organs and their internal innervation. The computer-aided portrayal sets new standards for the future. The succinct text clearly outlines what we already know and what remains to be discovered.

The same is true for all the other chapters. Particular mention should be made of the unrivalled depth of focus of the photographs and Gottfried Müller's excellent illustrations.

In contrast to other books on this topic, a chapter is dedicated to the prevention and management of complications.

The editors and authors are to be congratulated on a splendid volume. The effort invested in anatomical studies, illustrations and animal experiments exceeds by far that in other comparable titles.

Mainz, March 2007

R. Hohenfellner

Preface

Endoscopic/laparoscopic extraperitoneal radical prostatectomy has been established in the literature as an intriguing therapeutic option for the management of carcinoma of the prostate. Endoscopic and robotic approaches have proved to be equally effective for the management of localized prostate cancer. Nerve-sparing endoscopic/laparoscopic and robotic radical prostatectomy should aim to maintain sexual function and restore continence early after surgery without impairing the final oncological outcome.

The advent of laparoscopy and robotics has revitalized the discussion pertaining to the anatomy of the structures surrounding the prostate gland. Despite the different approaches for radical prostatectomy the key to better results is full understanding of the anatomy of the prostate, the bladder neck and the urethra. A special chapter has thus been devoted to the anatomy of the prostate and its surrounding structures.

There is a plethora of urology textbooks describing laparoscopic procedures in different ways. The present book is more an atlas than a conventional textbook. Our main goal is to guide the urologist step by step through the procedure, aiming to make this highly standardized technique reproducible. Every procedure is presented with numerous endoscopic images and diagrams so that the reader can fully comprehend the different surgical steps. Complications and useful tips and tricks for their management are described in detail.

We would like to thank Jens Mondry and Gottfried Müller for their significant contributions with regard to computer imaging and design creation, respectively. Furthermore, we would like to express our gratitude to all contributing authors for their significant scientific input.

Jens-Uwe Stolzenburg
Matthew T. Gettman
Evangelos N. Liatsikos

Contents

List of Contributors

Aedtner, Bernd, Dr. med.
Department of Anaesthesiology
and Intensive Care Medicine
University of Leipzig
Liebigstraße 20
04103 Leipzig, Germany

Anderson, Chris, MD
Consultant , Department of Urology
St Georges Hospital
London, UK

Bhanot, Shiv Mohan, MD
Consultant , Department of Urology
King George Hospital
London, UK

Dietel, Anja, Dr. med.
Department of Urology
University of Leipzig
Liebigstraße 20
04103 Leipzig, Germany

Do, Hoang Minh, Dr. med.
Department of Urology
University of Leipzig
Liebigstraße 20
04103 Leipzig, Germany

Filos, Kritos, MD
Associate Professor, Department of Anaesthesiology
and Intensive Care Medicine
University of Patras
26500 Rio, Patras, Greece

Gettman, Matthew T., MD
Associate Professor
Department of Urology
Mayo Clinic
Gonda 7S, 200 1st Street SW
Rochester, MN 55905, USA

Ho, Kossen, MD
Hong Kong Urology Clinic
510 Central Building, Pedder Street
Hong Kong, China

Hoffmann, Susanne, Dr. med.
Clinic Quellental
Wiesenweg 6
34537 Bad Wildungen, Germany

Hoffmann, W., Dr. med.
Clinic Quellental
Wiesenweg 6
34537 Bad Wildungen, Germany

Hohenfellner, Rudolf, Prof. Dr. med. em.
Department of Urology
University of Mainz
Saarstraße 21
55122 Mainz, Germany

Horn, Lars-Christian, Prof. Dr. med.
Institute of Pathology
University of Leipzig
Liebigstraße 13
04103 Leipzig, Germany

John, Hubert Andreas, PD Dr. med.
Department of Urology
Clinic Hirslanden
Witellikerstraße 40
8008 Zürich, Switzerland

Jünemann, Klaus-Peter, Prof. Dr. med.
Chairman, Department of Urology
University of Kiel
Olshausenstraße 40
24118 Kiel, Germany

Kallidonis, Panagiotis, MD
Department of Urology
University of Patras
26500 Rio, Patras, Greece

Katsakiori, Paraskevi, MD
Department of Urology
University of Patras
26500 Rio, Patras, Greece

König, Fritjoff, Prof. Dr. med.
Department of Anaesthesiology
and Intensive Care Medicine
University of Leipzig
Liebigstraße 20
04103 Leipzig, Germany

Kusche, Dirk, Dr. med.
Department of Urology
Klinikum Dortmund gGmbH
Beurhausstraße 40
44137 Dortmund, Germany

Liatsikos, Evangelos N., MD, PhD
Assistant Professor
Department of Urology
University of Patras
26500 Rio, Patras, Greece

Loeffler, Sabine, Dr. rer. nat.
Institute of Anatomy
University of Leipzig
Liebigstraße 13
04103 Leipzig, Germany

Luedtke, Torsten
Olympus Optical Co. (Europa) GmbH
Wendenstraße 14–18
20097 Hamburg, Germany

McNeil, Alan, BmedSci, FRCS (Ed & Eng), FRCS (Urol)
Consultant, Department of Urology
Western General Hospital
Crewe Road
Edinburgh, EH4 2XU, UK

Neuhaus, Jochen, Dr. rer. nat.
Department of Urology
University of Leipzig
Liebigstraße 20
04103 Leipzig, Germany

Otto, U., Prof. Dr. med.
Clinic Quellental
Wiesenweg 6
34537 Bad Wildungen, Germany

Papadoukakis, Stefanos, MD
Department of Urology
Klinikum Dortmund gGmbH
Beurhausstraße 40
44137 Dortmund, Germany

Pfeiffer, Heidemarie, Dr. med.
Department of Urology
University of Leipzig
Liebigstraße 20
04103 Leipzig, Germany

Rabenalt, Robert, Dr. med.
Department of Urology
University of Leipzig
Liebigstraße 20
04103 Leipzig, Germany

Schwaibold, Hartwig, Dr. med.
Chairman, Department of Urology
Kliniken am Steinenberg
Steinenbergstraße 25
72764 Reutlingen, Germany

Schwalenberg, Thilo, Dr. med.
Department of Urology
University of Leipzig
Liebigstraße 20
04103 Leipzig, Germany

Senet, Christine
Olympus Optical Co. (Europa) GmbH
Wendenstraße 14–18
20097 Hamburg, Germany

Sivalingam, Sivaprakasam, MD
Southmead Hospital
Bristol, UK

Spanel-Borowski, Katharina, Prof. Dr. med.
Chairman, Institute of Anatomy
University of Leipzig
Liebigstraße 13
04103 Leipzig, Germany

Stolzenburg, Jens-Uwe, Prof. Dr. med.
Chairman, Department of Urology
Head of International Training Centre
of Urologic Laparoscopy
University of Leipzig
Liebigstraße 20
04103 Leipzig, Germany

Truss, Michael C. , Prof. Dr. med.
Chairman, Department of Urology
Klinikum Dortmund gGmbH
Beurhausstraße 40
44137 Dortmund, Germany

Wehner, Markus, Dr. med.
Department of Anaesthesiology
and Intensive Care Medicine
University of Leipzig
Liebigstraße 20
04103 Leipzig, Germany

Winkler, Matthias, MD
Consultant, Department of Urology
Chairing Cross Hospital
Fulham Palace Road
London, W6 8RF, UK

List of Abbreviations

a	external iliac artery		**pc**	prostatic capsule
aw	abdominal wall		**pf**	periprostatic fascia
bl	bladder		**pg**	prostate glands
bm	bladder mucosa		**pl**	puboprostatic ligament
bn	bladder neck		**pln**	pelvic lymph nodes
bo	bladder outlet		**pp**	prostate pedicle
bp	bulb of penis		**pt**	peritoneum
bu	bulbourethalis glands (Cowper's glands)		**r**	rectum
ca	common iliac artery		**rm**	rectus muscle
dl	detrusor lamellae		**sc**	spermatic cord
dv	Denonvillier's fascia		**sp**	Santorini plexus
ef	endopelvic fascia		**sv**	seminal vesicle
ev	epigastric vessels		**u**	urethra
ia	internal iliac artery		**ul**	urethral lumen
iv	internal iliac vein		**ur**	ureter
la	levator ani muscle		**us**	urethral sphincter
nvb	neurovascular bundle		**v**	external iliac vein
oe	obturator externus muscle		**va**	(superior) vesical artery
oi	obturator internus muscle		**vd**	vas deferens
p	prostate		**vs**	vesical sphincter
pb	pubic bone			

History of Laparoscopy, Endoscopic Extraperitoneal Radical Prostatectomy and Robotic Surgery

1

Contents

Historical Aspects of Laparoscopy and Endoscopic Extraperitoneal Radical Prostatectomy

1.1

Stefanos Papadoukakis · Dirk Kusche · Michael C. Truss

1.1.1 History of Laparoscopy

"Laparoscopy" is derived from two Greek words meaning "flank" and "insight." Laparoscopy is the established term although „celioscopy", meaning intraabdominal insight, would have been more accurate. Today "laparoscopy" describes a procedure during which contents of the intraperitoneal cavity or of the extraperitoneal space are examined and manipulated in a diagnostic or therapeutic intervention.

Although the term has been widely used in urology only in the past 15 years, the concept is actually more than 100 years old. It was at the beginning of the 20th century that Kelling experimentally insufflated the abdominal cavity of a dog and inserted a cystoscope to inspect the abdominal visceral organs [6] (Figs. 1.1.1, 1.1.2).

Urology began to embrace laparoscopy as an essential diagnostic procedure in the early 1970s. By that time urologists had started using laparoscopy to search for undescended cryptorchid testes that were entrapped in the abdominal cavity, anywhere along their route from the retroperitoneal space to the scrotum.

The status of laparoscopy in urology did not change dramatically in the following decade and it was always a diagnostic procedure only. It was not until the 1990s that two reports described another, more advanced use of laparoscopy in our specialty.

Clayman et al., in 1991, reported the first laparoscopically performed nephrectomy with simultaneous intracorporeal tissue morcellation and use of impermeable specimen sacs to permit organ removal through the endoscopic ports [2]. Some doubted whether morcellation of the kidney was an adequate method for organ removal in an oncologic setting. The first hand-assisted nephrectomy was described by Nakada and colleagues in 1997 and this has remained an alternative approach to radical nephrectomy [7]. Nowadays, radical nephrectomy has become

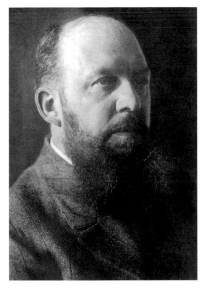

Fig. 1.1.1 Georg Kelling (1866–1945): the man who introduced modern laparoscopy into medicine

the standard approach due to ongoing technical and technological refinements in laparoscopy.

Almost at the same time, Schuessler et al. reported the first laparoscopically performed lymphadenectomy for prostate cancer [10]. For many urologists, this procedure was the first and most intriguing insight into the world of laparoscopy.

Laparoscopic ligation of the spermatic veins for varicocele is a widely performed procedure and a good training opportunity to help urologists familiarize themselves with the laparoscopic instruments and the laparoscopic reality. The translation of the two-dimensional monitor picture into three-dimensional movement of the surgeon's hands has a certain learning curve, and varicocele ligation is considered as an "entry" or training procedure for more complex operations.

1

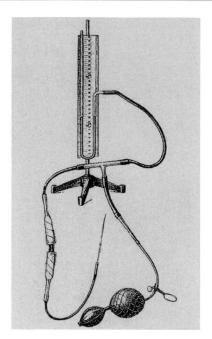

Fig. 1.1.2 The Kelling apparatus (cystoscope with insufflation to inspect the abdominal cavity in a dog

The modern laparoscopic era has evolved dramatically over the course of the past decade. It is a worldwide reality that almost every single urologic operation, oncologic or otherwise, can be performed laparoscopically just as efficiently, and with fewer and less serious complications, as with conventional open surgery. UPJ reconstruction, retroperitoneal lymphadenectomy, radical nephrectomy with vena cava thrombus extraction, live donor nephrectomy during renal transplantation, radical prostatectomy, even radical cystectomy with continent diversion – from minor to major operations, urologists have managed to incorporate laparoscopy into everyday urologic practice. The future is promising and exciting. The advent of robotic technologies and robot-assisted surgery, with and without tactile feedback, is already a reality in modern urological practice. Nevertheless, there is currently not enough evidence to show that these techniques indeed provide advantages over "conventional" laparoscopy, either in functional or in oncological outcomes. Furthermore, it has not yet been possible to demonstrate that robot-assisted surgery is cost effective.

1.1.2 Laparoscopic Radical Prostatectomy

As mentioned above, Schuessler and coworkers were the first to perform laparoscopic lymphadenectomy for prostate cancer prior to open radical prostatectomy [10]. The same group described removal of the seminal vesicles during laparoscopic lymphadenectomy [5]. In 1992 this group was the first to perform transperitoneal laparoscopic radical prostatectomies, and they published their initial series of 9 patients in 1997 [9]. They were not enthusiastic about the technique and concluded that "...laparoscopy is not an efficacious surgical alternative to open prostatectomy for malignancy...." This team was not able to define a clear advantage of laparoscopic surgery over the traditional open radical retropubic prostatectomy regarding hospital stay, continence and reconvalescence. It is noteworthy that these first operations lasted almost 9 h on average, which was considered a major drawback for the further development of the technique.

Raboy et al. described the first extraperitoneal radical prostatectomy and, in contrast to the Schuessler group, they were rather satisfied with the results of the new evolving technique [8].

In December 1997 Guilloneau and colleagues performed a transperitoneal laparoscopic radical prostatectomy in less than 6 h, and in January 1998 the same team started to perform their first series of laparoscopic radical prostatectomy [3, 4]. Laparoscopic radical prostatectomy soon became a widespread minimally invasive alternative to radical prostatectomy, so that by the year 2001 more than 1,200 radical prostatectomies had been performed, mainly in European centers. Ever since then a rapidly increasing number of urologic departments, both in Europe and the USA, have performed large series of this innovative minimally invasive technique. Many urologists have suggested various modifications of the original operation, including transperitoneal or extraperitoneal approach, antegrade or retrograde dissection and different neurovascular bundle-sparing techniques.

Over the past few years, laparoscopic radical prostatectomy has become the standard procedure for the treatment of localized prostate cancer in an increasing number of urologic centers in Europe and in the USA.

The well-known advantages of minimally invasive surgery over conventional open surgery have led to increasing interest worldwide in the further development of laparoscopy in urology. These benefits include less postoperative pain, a shorter hospital stay, and faster resumption of normal activities along with a minimally invasive technique that provides better visualization of the operative field through the optic magnification, shorter catheterization time and minimal intraoperative blood loss. To the aforementioned advantages we have to add the fact that laparoscopic radical prostatectomy is oncologically just as efficient as the traditional open retropubic prostatectomy and has similar or better functional results in experienced hands.

In a recent survey in Germany, 35% of laparoscopically active departments already performed laparoscopic prostatectomy and almost all of the rest intended to introduce in the near future [19].

1.1.3 Extraperitoneal Access – The Term "EERPE"

The first laparoscopic prostatectomies described were performed using transperitoneal access. Despite the fact that the extraperitoneal route was almost simultaneously reported [8], the French team at the Montsouris center chose to develop the transperitoneal approach [4].

The groups in France refined and evolved the technique and reduced operation time to 3–4 h, not much more than a third of the time initially reported by Schuessler. Later on the French experience spread throughout Europe.

However, general skepticism persisted due to the fact that an extraperitoneal organ, the prostate, was being accessed by a transperitoneal route with possible intraperitoneal complications: bowel injuries, intraperitoneal bleeding, ileus, intraperitoneal leakage of urine, and acute infection of the peritoneal cavity are considered the main short-term or intraoperative complications, while intraperitoneal adhesion formation and subsequent chronic bowel obstruction with recurrent ileus are the principal long-term complications.

The perspective of an extraperitoneal approach to the prostate was developed after the initial report by Raboy and coworkers. The first series of 42 patients to undergo extraperitoneal radical prostatectomy was published by Bollens et al. in 2001 [1].

The extraperitoneal approach to radical prostatectomy bears the advantages of a minimally invasive technique for the removal of the prostate while overcoming the limitations of a transperitoneal approach (i.e., potential problems in visualization, and increased risk of intra- and postoperative intraperitoneal complications).

A further development of the technique was reported by Stolzenburg et al. as EERPE in 2002 [11]. The term endoscopic extraperitoneal radical prostatectomy (EERPE) was used to describe the totally extraperitoneal access to the prostate for radical prostatectomy. Based on the growing experience with this technique, the same group has proposed many modifications and improvements of this operation, including a standardized and reproducible nerve-sparing, potency-preserving approach [18]. Furthermore, preservation of the puboprostatic ligaments for better early postoperative continence rates, minimal blood loss, and the reliable oncologic results (regarding positive margins) have made this approach the standard and first option for the treatment of localized prostate cancer in many specialized centers [13, 14]. EERPE is an ever-evolving procedure. The latest technique involves intrafascial preparation of the prostate leaving the pelvic fascias intact [15]. This approach reflects the latest anatomical studies identifying neurovascular structures not only dorsolateral to the prostate but also within the prostatic fascia laterally and anterolaterally.

In contrast to "traditional" thinking, there are almost no limiting factors for minimally invasive radical prostatectomy and especially for EERPE. Previous abdominal or pelvic surgery, for example, is no barrier. Modifications of trocar placement and operative techniques have made EERPE possible even for patients considered unsuitable for minimally invasive surgery in the past [12, 16, 17].

It is of paramount importance to point out that the evolution of the technique has been assisted by advances in medical equipment and instruments. In the past few years the development of devices such as endoscopic clip applicators, harmonic scalpels and endoscopic multiple-use instruments, as well as two-component sealants, has promoted minimal invasive surgery in urology.

Today it is clear that EERPE has already reached (if not, indeed, surpassed) the standards of open radical prostatectomy. One of the major problems that many urologists face is the long and steep learning curve of laparoscopic procedures. Therefore, a new modular training concept has been developed for EERPE in order to standardize the surgical training and shorten the learning curve of both laparoscopically experienced and laparoscopically naive surgeons [16].

In summary, today EERPE is a first-line option for patients with localized prostate cancer in a rapidly increasing number of urologic departments around the globe. Innovative developments such as EERPE, together with cutting-edge technological advances, enable urology to remain in the forefront of medical and technical development.

References

1. Bollens R, Van den Bosche M, Roumeguere T et al (2001) Extraperitoneal laparoscopic radical prostatectomy: results after 50 cases. Eur Urol 40:65–69
2. Clayman RV, Kavoussi LR, Sopper NJ et al (1991) Laparoscopic nephrectomy: initial case report. J Urol 146:278
3. Guilloneau B, Vallancien G (2000) Laparoscopic radical prostatectomy: the Montsouris technique. J Urol 163:1643
4. Guilloneau B, Rozet F, Cathelineau X, Vallancien G et al (2002) Perioperative complications of laparoscopic radical prostatectomy: the Montsouris 3 year experience. J Urol 167:51–56
5. Kavoussi LR, Schuessler WW, VancaillieTG, Clayman RV (1993) Laparoscopic approach to the seminal vesicles. J Urol 150:417–419
6. Kelling G (1923) Zur Colioskopie. Arch Clin Chir 126:226
7. Nakada SY, Moon TD, Gist M et al (1997) Use of a Pneumo Sleeve as an adjunct in laparoscopic nephrectomy. Urology 49:612
8. Raboy A, Ferzli G, Albert P (1997) Initial experience with extraperitoneal endoscope radical retropubic prostatectomy. Urology 50:849–853
9. Schuessler WW, Schulam PG, Clayman RV et al (1997) Laparoscopic radical prostatectomy: initial short term experience. Urology 50:854
10. Schuessler WW, Vancaillie TG, Reich H et al (1991) Transperitoneal endosurgical lymphadenectomy in patients with localized prostate cancer. J Urol 145:988
11. Stolzenburg JU, Do M, Pfeiffer H et al (2002) The endoscopic extraperitoneal radical prostatectomy (EERPE): technique and initial experience. World J Urol 20:48–55
12. Stolzenburg JU, Ho K, Do M, Rabenalt R, Dorschner W, Truss M (2005) Impact of previous surgery on endoscopic extraperitoneal radical prostatectomy. Urology 65:325–331
13. Stolzenburg JU, Liatsikos EN, Rabenalt R, Do M, Sakelaropoulos G, Horn LC, Truss MC (2006) Nerve sparing endoscopic extraperitoneal radical prostatectomy – effect of puboprostatic ligament preservation on early continence and positive margins. Eur Urol 49:103–112
14. Stolzenburg JU, Rabenalt R, Do M, Ho K, Dorschner W, Waldkirch E, Jonas U, Schützt A, Horn L, Truss M (2005) Endoscopic extraperitoneal radical prostatectomy: oncological and functional results after 700 procedures. J Urol 174:1271–1275
15. Stolzenburg JU, Rabenalt R, Tannapfel A, Liatsikos E (2006) Intrafascial nerve sparing endoscopic extraperitoneal radical prostatectomy. Urology 67:17–21
16. Stolzenburg JU, Schwaibold H, Bhanot S, Rabenalt R, Do M, Truss M, Ho K, Anderson C (2005) Modular surgical training for endoscopic extraperitoneal radical prostatectomy. BJU Int 96:1022–1027
17. Stolzenburg JU, Truss M, Bekos A, Do M, Rabenalt M, Stief C, Hoznek A, Abbou CC, Neuhaus J, Dorschner W (2004) Does the extraperitoneal laparoscopic approach improve the outcome of radical prostatectomy? Curr Urol Rep 5:115–122
18. Stolzenburg JU, Truss MC, Do M, Rabenalt R, Pfeiffer H, Dunzinger M, Aedtner, Stief CG, Jonas U, Dorschner W (2003) Evolution of endoscopic extraperitoneal radical prostatectomy (EERPE) – technical improvements and development of a nerve-sparing, potency-preserving approach. World J Urol 21:147–152
19. Vogeli TA, Burchard M, Fornara P et al (2002) Laparoscoping working group of the German Urological Association. Current laparoscopic practice patterns in urology: results of a survey among urologists in Germany and Switzerland. Eur Urol 42:441–446

Historical Overview of Robotic Radical Prostatectomy

Matthew T. Gettman · Hubert John

The development of minimally invasive laparoscopic techniques has had a profound impact on urology in the past decade. Despite the numerous patient-related advantages of many minimally invasive procedures, laparoscopic techniques are often more difficult to perform than corresponding tasks in open surgery. Indeed, the technical learning curve for minimally invasive laparoscopic techniques can be very steep. Laparoscopy can impose limitations on instrument manipulation (secondary to trocar positioning), dexterity (secondary to long non-articulated instruments), tissue palpation (lack of haptic interface), and vision (two-dimensional on flat screen). Robotic surgery has been developed to increase operative precision, decrease the learning curve, and thereby increase clinical applicability of minimally invasive laparoscopic techniques. Since the introduction of surgical robots, a rapid technologic evolution has been witnessed in urology [1, 2].

The first clinically available surgical robot in urology was purposely designed to hold a laparoscope [3]. This robot, called the Automated Endoscope System for Optimal Positioning (AESOP, Intuitive Surgical, Sunnyvale, CA), has one robotic arm with six degrees of freedom (DOF) that is directly mounted on the operating table [3, 4]. The robot is controlled using a foot pedal, joystick, or voice commands. Kavoussi et al. noted that AESOP improved image quality and eliminated the need for surgical assistants during a variety of laparoscopic procedures, including ureterolysis, pelvic lymphadenectomy, nephrectomy, and pyeloplasty [3]. Recently, Antiphon et al. demonstrated the feasibility of laparoscopic radical prostatectomy (RP) performed with the use of a single surgeon, self-retaining retractors, and AESOP [5]. The introduction of AESOP also facilitated the development of telementoring and teleproctoring, which have also made laparoscopic surgery more applicable [6].

Building on the foundations of the AESOP robot, more advanced robotics systems have been introduced clinically within the past 5 years. These robots were derived from experimental robotic systems developed in the early 1990s [7, 8]. More advanced robots, also known as master–slave robots, have a remote control unit that is used to control multiple robotic instruments and camera arms. Using master–slave robots, surgeons use hand controls to maneuver three or four mechanical arms placed inside the patient [1, 2]. All surgical movements are enhanced and replicated by the robot. For instance, the robot can potentially improve performance by filtering away physiologic tremors. One of the first systems was introduced by Bowersox and Cornum for open surgery [7]. The system used three-dimensional imaging and interchangeable surgical instruments positioned on two mechanical arms. Another innovative telerobot with tactile feedback (i.e. haptic interface) was similarly introduced by Schurr et al. with favorable experimental results [8].

From a historical standpoint, the Zeus robot (Intuitive Surgical, Sunnyvale, CA) was one of the first master–slave robots to be introduced clinically [1, 2]. When initially introduced, the robot lacked three-dimensional vision capability as well as articulated instrumentation. Given the design deficiencies, another robotics system called da Vinci has emerged as the leading telerobot to date in the operating room.

The da Vinci robotic system (Intuitive Surgical, Mountain View, CA) is also a master–slave robot that includes two or three robotic instrument arms, a camera arm, a standard three-dimensional imaging system, and a remote control unit [1, 2]. Since FDA approval of the initial da Vinci robot, more advanced versions of this system have been introduced [9]. For example, the so-called fourth-arm da Vinci robot reduces reliance on assistants when performing robotic surgery. The latest robot, called the da Vinci S, incorporates the fourth-arm features as well as other features to potentially make the system easier to use for the surgeon and assistants.

Using a da Vinci robot, manipulator arms are attached to the patient via reusable laparoscopic ports and the camera arm is placed through a standard trocar [1, 2]. Da Vinci instruments have limited reusability, but are designed to replicate wrist motions by providing six DOF and grip. Over the years, da Vinci instrumentation has improved substantially to more closely parallel instruments used in pure laparoscopic or open surgery. Images with da Vinci are viewed with high magnification, but da Vinci systems lack a force-feedback feature, require cumbersome robotic installation, can impair intraoperative communication, and are associated with high financial cost. In part, the additional costs of da Vinci are related to required use of interchangeable instruments with limited reusability [10]. Upon attaching the instrument to the robotic arm, the system automatically subtracts „life" from the instrument.

Similar to conventional laparoscopy, a learning curve is also present with telerobotics. The robotic learning curve is thought, however, to be much less steep than that of conventional laparoscopy [1, 2]. Technical factors that must be overcome include operating preferentially with visual cues and operating with high magnification. The learning curve is also related to the teamwork between the remotely seated surgeon and the assistants sterilely scrubbed at the operating table.

Robotic surgical techniques have been developed experimentally and clinically for a wide variety of applications in the upper and lower urinary tract [11–19]. Although telerobotic nephrectomies and adrenalectomies have been reported, robotic indications in the upper tract have favored reconstructive versus extirpative procedures. Since the clinical description in 2002, robotic pyeloplasty has been increasingly performed for ureteropelvic junction obstruction [15]. In the lower urinary tract, telerobots are most commonly utilized for RP, but other procedures such as radical cystectomy and urinary diversion are gaining momentum [16, 17].

Initial experience with da Vinci for laparoscopic RP was described predominantly at centers with significant experience in non-robotic laparoscopic RP or open RP [11, 18–20]. Since that time, interest in robotic prostatectomy has increased exponentially. The technique of robotic prostatectomy is standardized using either a transperitoneal or an extraperitoneal approach [11, 18–20]. Data comparing the results of da Vinci RP, open RP, and pure laparoscopic RP suggest that the robotic technique is at the very least equivalent to the other techniques at short-term follow-up [19]. Ongoing evaluation of outcomes data is required to further understand the clinical advantages of robotic prostatectomy in comparison to other prostatectomy techniques.

In summary, robotic surgery has rapidly developed in urology. For many urologic problems in the upper and lower urinary tract, a standardized approach with a surgical robot is considered a bona fide treatment option. At the present time, robotic surgery in urology is most commonly used for RP. The technique is increasingly being successfully embraced by surgeons with or without prior experience in laparoscopy using either a transperitoneal or an extraperitoneal approach. Longer follow-up and analysis of outcomes data is needed to confidently determine safety of all robotic procedures. Nonetheless, robotics does appear established in urology and is expected to continue to have a favorable evolution and impact on future generations of surgeons with improved telecommunications, imaging, computer technologies, miniaturization, and the advent of virtual reality.

References

1. Gettman MT, Blute ML, Peschel R, Bartsch G (2003) Current status of robotics in urologic laparoscopy. Eur Urol 43:106–112
2. Gettman MT, Cadeddu JA (2004) Robotics in urologic surgery. In: Graham SD (ed) Glenn's urologic surgery, 6th edn. Lippincott Williams & Wilkins, Philadelphia, pp 1027–1033
3. Kavoussi LR, Moore RG, Partin AW, Bender JS, Zenilman ME, Satava RM (1994) Telerobotic assisted laparoscopic surgery: initial laboratory and clinical experience. Urology 44:15–19
4. Partin AW, Adams JB, Moore RG, Kavoussi LR (1995) Complete robot-assisted laparoscopic urologic surgery: a preliminary report. J Am Coll Surg 181:552–557
5. Antiphon P, Hoznek A, Benyoussef A, et al (2003) Complete solo laparoscopic radical prostatectomy: initial experience. Urology 61:724
6. Janetschek G, Bartsch G, Kavoussi LR (1998) Transcontinental interactive laparoscopic telesurgery between the United States and Europe. J Urol 160:1413
7. Bowersox JC, Cornum RL (1998) Remote operative urology using a surgical telemanipulator system: preliminary observations. Urology 52:17–22

8. Schurr MO, Buess G, Neisius B (2000) Robotics and tele-manipulation technologies for endoscopic surgery: a review of the ARTEMIS project. Surg Endosc 14:375–381

9. Esposito MP, Ilbeigi P, Ahmed M, Lanteri V (2005) Use of fourth arm in daVinci robot-assisted extraperitoneal laparoscopic prostatectomy: novel technique. Urology 66:649–652

10. Lotan Y, Cadeddu JA, Gettman MT (2004) The new economics of radical prostatectomy: cost comparison of open, laparoscopic and robot assisted techniques. J Urol 172:1431–1435

11. Abbou CC, Hoznek A, Salomon L, Olsson LE, Lobontiu A, Saint F, Cicco A, Antiphon P, Chopin D (2001) Laparoscopic radical prostatectomy with remote controlled robot. J Urol 165:1964–1966

12. Gill IS, Sung GT, Hsu TH, Meraney AM (2000) Robotic remote laparoscopic nephrectomy and adrenalectomy: initial experience. J Urol 164:2082–2085

13. Guillonneau B, Jayet C, Tewari A, Vallancien G (2001) Robot assisted laparoscopic nephrectomy. J Urol 166:200–201

14. Bentas W, Wolfram M, Brautigam R, Binder J (2002) Laparoscopic transperitoneal adrenalectomy using a remote controlled robotic surgical system. J Endourol 16:373–376

15. Gettman MT, Neururer R, Bartsch G, Peschel R (2002) Anderson-Hynes dismembered pyeloplasty performed using the daVinci robotic system. Urology 60:509–513

16. Hubert J, Chammas M, Larre S, et al (2006) Initial experience with successful totally robotic laparoscopic cysto-prostatectomy and ileal conduit construction in tetraplegic patient: report of two cases. J Endourol 20:139–143

17. Shah NL, Hemal AK, Menon M (2005) Robot-assisted radical cystectomy and urinary diversion. Curr Urol Rep 6:122–125

18. Binder J, Kramer W (2001) Robotically-assisted laparoscopic radical prostatectomy. BJU Int 87:408–410

19. Menon M, Tewari A, Baize B, Guillonneau B, Vallancien G (2002) Prospective comparison of radical retropubic prostatectomy and robot-assisted anatomic prostatectomy: the Vattikuti Urology Institute experience. Urology 60:864–868

20. Gettman MT, Hoznek A, Salomon L, et al (2003) Laparoscopic radical prostatectomy: description of the extraperitoneal approach using the daVinci robotic system. J Urol 170:416–419

Surgical Anatomy
for Radical Prostatectomy

2

Contents

Surgical Neuroanatomy of the Male Pelvis

2.1

Thilo Schwalenberg · Rudolph Hohenfellner · Jochen Neuhaus · Mathias H. Winkler
Evangelos N. Liatsikos · Jens-Uwe Stolzenburg

Exact neuroanatomical knowledge of the male and female pelvis has become increasingly important to both anatomists and pelvic surgeons (bowel surgery, urology, gynaecology). Anatomical discoveries are often the basis for the development of new operating methods. In addition, functional results after operative procedures have become the target of detailed anatomical scrutiny.

New operating methods that spare the important neural structures of the urogenital tract have led to improved results in terms of bladder function, urinary continence and erectile potency. Well-described examples are nerve-sparing radical prostatectomy [1, 2] and cystectomy [2, 3] (continence, potency), ureteric antireflux surgery [4] (bladder function), extended radical hysterectomy with total mesometrial resection [5, 6] (bladder function) and rectal resection [7, 8] (continence, bladder function, potency).

Urologists, gynaecologists and bowel surgeons often encounter neural structures of similar origin in the true pelvis. Commonly, visceral pelvic nerves of organs dealt with by one specialty run through the operating spaces of another specialty. This requires an interdisciplinary approach. A new generation of pelvic surgeons is called for.

2.1.1 Neuroanatomical Basics of Radical Prostatectomy

During radical prostatectomy the surgeon encounters nerve fibres that run dorsally and laterally to the prostate, also known as neurovascular bundles (NVB). This term does not have an exact anatomical correlate as it describes a topographically related cluster of nerves and blood vessels. In the literature the description of the NVB differs widely and in regard to its existence and exact position is subject to inter-individual variations [9–12]. These autonomic nerve fibres

originate in the pelvic plexus (synonyms: pelvic ganglion, inferior hypogastric plexus), which unites sympathetic and parasympathetic nerves. In contrast to the NVB the pelvic plexus is an anatomical structure subjected to only minute inter-individual variability. It is rhombic in shape, situated at the lateral pelvic wall and represents a concentration of ganglion cells. The pelvic plexus is the central neural plexus that provides autonomic innervation to male urogenital organs. Particular attention is paid to the dissection and preservation of nerves that run from the NVB to the cavernosal bodies during radical prostatectomy. These purely autonomic nerves are called nervi cavernosi penis (or cavernosal nerves).

The autonomic supply is strictly separated from somatosensory nerves. The relevant nerve in regard to radical prostatectomy is the pudendal nerve, which supplies not only the muscles for erection and ejaculation but also the striated part of the external urethral sphincter. Especially during apical dissection, potential for injury exists at radical prostatectomy.

With regard to the neuroanatomy of radical prostatectomy the discussion here focuses on the localisation of the NVB, the question of autonomic innervation of urethral sphincter structures and the existence of nerve connections between autonomic and somatosensory systems. Historically, the discussion about neural structures concerned with continence and erectile function began as early as 1863, when Eckhard [13] defined the nervi erigentes in animal experiments. In a landmark paper in 1982, Walsh and Donker [14] highlighted the clinical relevance of cavernosal nerves for the preservation of potency at radical prostatectomy.

Table 2.1.1 shows historically important publications which have profoundly influenced our understanding and surgical methodology in the quest for preservation of autonomic pelvic nerves.

Table 2.1.1. Important historical publications on the neuroanatomy of the pelvis

Publication	Summary
Müller 1835 [15]	Detailed anatomic drawings of autonomic fibres within pelvis; distinction of sympathetic and parasympathetic portions as well as fibres supplying penis and as a result of their proximity to lateral surface of prostate, description of a plexus prostaticus; demarcation of pudendal nerve
Budge 1858 [16]	First experimental investigations with electrical stimulation of hypogastric nerve in animals and measurement of response at ejaculatory duct and seminal vesicles
Eckhard 1863 [13]	Experimental investigations and description of relationship between pelvic plexus and erection in animals; definition of nervi erigentes as main parasympathetic nerves for erection
Calabrisi 1955 [17]	Survey of origin of cavernosal nerves and description of their anatomic pathway in foetal and embryonal state
Davis and Jelenko 1975 [8]	Reflections on sexual changes in patients after abdominoperineal resection; discussion of protection of pelvic plexus to preserve postoperative sexual function
Walsh and Donker 1982 [14]	Description of neurovascular bundle, coinage of term anatomical radical prostatectomy with protection of dorsolaterally localised neurovascular bundle; first definition of a valid operational standard
Lue et al. 1984 [18]	Comparative nerve topography of erection by means of cadaveric dissection in animal and man
Lepor et al. 1985 [9]	Detailed nerve topography and precise relationship of cavernosal nerves of pelvic plexus to urethra, lateral pelvic fascia, prostatic capsule and Denonvilliers' fascia
Schlegel and Walsh 1987 [3]	Importance of neurovascular bundle preservation at radical cystectomy
Jünemann et al. 1988 [19]	Sacral and pudendal plexus, differentiated investigations of sacral roots S2-S4
Fritsch 1989 [20]	Topography of pelvic plexus in foetal state (21–29 weeks); definition of pelvic connective tissues; study of fibre direction along urethral sphincter
Stelzner et al. 1989 [7]	Experience from potency-preserving rectal surgery; investigation of embryos and newborns; relationship between nervi erigentes, anterior rectal wall, pelvic floor and diaphragmatic part of urethra before entering two cavernosal bodies of penis; exact determination of nerve density at anterior rectal wall; preservation of sexual function, using own patient population
Breza et al. 1989 [21]	Cadaveric study on description of vascular anatomy, in particular at entrance to cavernosal bodies; proof of connections between dorsal nerve and cavernosal nerve of penis at level of crura penis
Stief et al. 1991 [22]	Role of sympathetic nervous system during erection
Paick et al. 1993 [23]	Study on adult cadavers with detailed description of autonomous nerve fibre direction distal to prostate up to entrance into cavernosal bodies; description of medial urethral branches of cavernosal nerve, interaction between cavernosal nerve and dorsal nerve of penis
Zvara et al. 1994 [24]	Detailed neuroanatomy of urethral sphincter, innervation of intrinsic and extrinsic segments of urethral sphincter by sacral segments S2–4 of pudendal nerve
Strasser and Bartsch 1996 [25]	Innervation of urethral sphincter (described as striated sphincter, „rhabdosphincter", by authors) by pudendal nerve, no role of cavernosal nerve and pelvic plexus; autonomous fibres of pelvic plexus run to membranous urethra
Höckel et al. 1998 [6]	Development of liposuction-assisted nerve-sparing extended radical hysterectomy to improve conventional gynaecological pelvic surgery and avoid urinary bladder dysfunction
Höer et al. 2000 [26]	Cadaveric study; detailed description of topography of autonomic nerves and their lesions in pelvic surgery; importance of a sympathetic lesion during high ligation of inferior mesenteric artery; discussion of differences in terminology of pelvic fascia and anatomical landmarks in pelvic surgery

2

Table 2.1.1. (continued)

Publication	Summary
Leißner et al. 2001 [4]	Accurate topography of pelvic plexus and related fibres on human cadavers fixed with Thiel solution; staining of nerves with methylene blue; description of lesions of pelvic plexus; clinical importance during antireflux surgery and trigonal reconstruction in prostate surgery; also refers to possible intraoperative use of methylene blue to identify autonomic nerves
Akita et al. 2003 [27]	Detailed cadaveric study on origin and anatomical pathway of nerves supplying urethral sphincter; innervation of urethral sphincter by pudendal nerve and pelvic plexus
Kiyoshima et al. 2004 [12]	Detailed investigations of periprostatic fibromuscular stroma regarding existence and course of fascial structures (Denonvilliers' fascia, laterally pelvic fascia) and nerve structures, preparations after non-nerve-sparing radical prostatectomy; a dorsolaterally located NVB was found in only 48% of cases, the NVB was separated by adipose tissue in 52% and neural structures were spread over lateral surface of prostate without 'classic' bundling
Costello et al. 2004 [11]	Detailed topography of NVB in cadavers; classification of NVB into three functional compartments (posterior/posterolateral – rectum; lateral – levator ani; anterior – prostate/cavernosal nerves); clinical importance for sural nerve graft interposition after sacrifice of cavernosal nerves during radical prostatectomy
Takenaka et al. 2005 [28]	Inter-individual variation in distribution of extramural ganglion cells in male pelvis; immunohistochemical differentiation into sympathetic and parasympathetic ganglia; description of autonomic cells not only in nerve components but also along viscera in coexistence with both cell types in a ganglion

2.1.2 Sympathetic System

Sympathetic fibres responsible for the innervation of the lower urinary tract and male genital organs arise from thoracolumbar segments T10–12 and L1–2. They leave the spinal column via the anterior rami of the spinal nerves and finally reach the sympathetic chain via communicating rami albi. Some fibres are relayed in the renal ganglia, which reach the testis and epididymus as testicular plexus. The main sympathetic effect at the end organ is vasoconstriction. Other sympathetic fibres reach the lumbar and sacral ganglia. These fibres arise from spinal segments L1–2 and are commonly known as lumbar and sacral splanchnic nerves. Splanchnic nerves communicate with anterior roots of spinal segments S2–4 after relay and run through the superior hypogastric plexus at level L3–S1, where they divide into paired hypogastric nerves, vesical, prostatic and deferential plexus, and a supply to the urethra.

The sympathetic innervation is responsible for the secretory functions of the prostate and seminal vesicles as well as ejaculation (contraction of the vas deferens and synchronous activation of the internal urethral sphincter). Hence, injury to the pelvic sympathetic fibres during extended lymphadenectomy of a radical cystectomy or retroperitoneal lymph node dissection for testicular cancer may cause retrograde ejaculation. The anatomical location of most pelvic sympathetic fibres is the superior hypogastric plexus after division of the left and right hypogastric nerves (Fig. 2.1.1).

2.1.3 Parasympathetic System

The sacral component of the parasympathetic system originates from spinal segments S2–4. Sacral fibres run in the spinal nerves of the pudendal plexus but emerge shortly after exit from the sacral foramina as pelvic splanchnic nerves (Fig. 2.1.2). Their further presynaptic course follows the rectum and the dorsolateral boundaries of the prostate. The relay station for sympathetic and parasympathetic fibres, which emerge as the important pelvic plexus, is also situated here. The pelvic plexus also receives the sympathetic hypogastric nerves, which form after division of the superior hypogastric plexus. This mesh of parasympathetic and sympathetic fibres gives rise caudally to the cavernosal nerves of the penis, which eventually innervate the cavernosal bodies. Figures 2.1.3 and

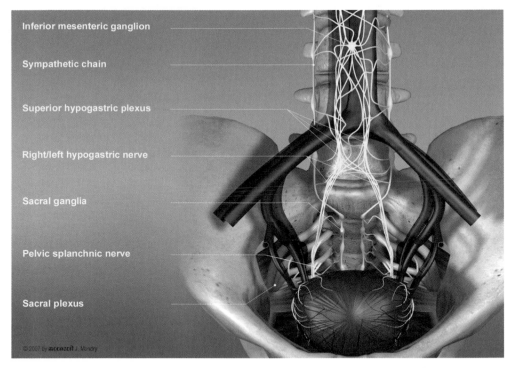

Fig. 2.1.1. Division of superior hypogastric plexus into paired hypogastric plexus for sympathetic supply of the pelvis

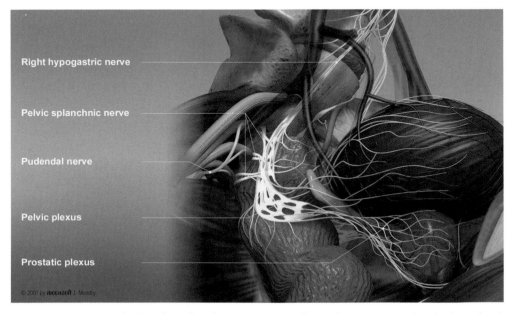

Fig. 2.1.2. Formation of pelvic plexus from hypogastric nerves (sympathetic component) and pelvic splanchnic nerves (parasympathetic component). Initially, sympathetic and parasympathetic fibres run together with fibres of the pudendal nerve in spinal roots S2–4

2

2.1.4 show that the cavernosal nerves of the penis traverse the apex of the prostate at a distance of only a few millimetres from the prostatic capsule at the 5 and 7 o'clock positions. Together with the deep artery and vein of the penis (A. et V. profunda penis), the cavernosal nerves of the penis enter the crura after exiting from the muscular pelvis. Stimulation of parasympathetic nerves leads to dilatation of smooth-muscle-lined cavernosal sinuses which effects influx of blood with subsequent tumescence. Hence, the parasympathetic system is the main neural component for erectile function.

2.1.4 Pelvic Plexus (Inferior Hypogastric Plexus, Pelvic Ganglion)

The pelvic plexus is a collection of ganglia which is located lateral to pelvic organs. It has a rhombic shape with a longitudinal diameter of ca. 5 centimetres and is located at the apex of the seminal vesicles.

In the male the plexus is situated laterally to the rectum, seminal vesicle, prostate and posterior part of the bladder (Fig. 2.1.2). These structures may be injured during radical cystectomy, rectal resection, ure-

teric antireflux surgery or extended radical hysterectomy (Wertheim's operation).

Sympathetic fibres of the superior hypogastric plexus, the sacral sympathetic chain ganglia and parasympathetic fibres of the pelvic splanchnic nerves, as well as somatic afferents, feed into the pelvic plexus. This is the main coordinating centre for pelvic autonomic innervation. The main efferent branches are the vesical plexus with fibres for the urinary bladder and the seminal vesicles; the prostatic plexus with fibres for the prostate, seminal vesicle, bulbourethral glands and ejaculatory ducts as well as cavernosal nerves for the cavernosal bodies; the deferential plexus for the vas deferens; the ureteric plexus for the pelvic ureter; and the medial and inferior rectal plexus with fibres for the colon and external anal sphincter muscle.

The nerve-sparing radical prostatectomy was developed to protect the pelvic plexus and the cavernosal nerves of the penis, which arise from the NVB. The nerve fibres of the NVB are of microscopic calibre and can only be recognised by the presence of the accompanying vascular structures. Accompanying arterial vessels arise from the prostatic arteries. Venous vessels channel into the prostatic venous plexus (Fig. 2.1.3).

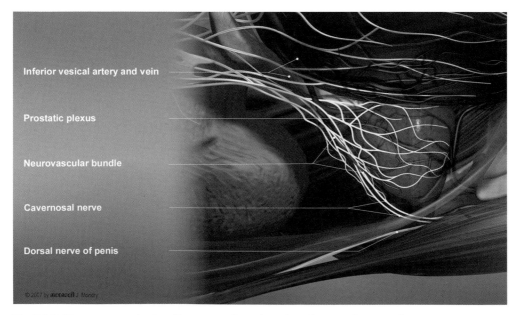

Inferior vesical artery and vein

Prostatic plexus

Neurovascular bundle

Cavernosal nerve

Dorsal nerve of penis

© 2007 by Michael J. Mondry

Fig. 2.1.3. The neurovascular bundle emerges from the pelvic plexus and its neural component continues distally as the cavernosal nerves of the penis. The prostatic plexus supplies the prostate. The pudendal nerve continues as the dorsal nerve of the penis and lies externally to the levator "hammock"

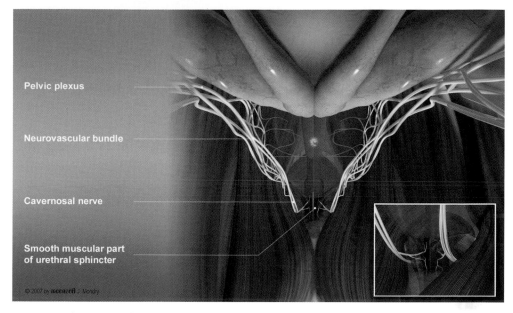

Pelvic plexus

Neurovascular bundle

Cavernosal nerve

Smooth muscular part
of urethral sphincter

© 2007 by sobotta J. Mondry

Fig. 2.1.4. The cavernosal nerves of the penis emerge from the neurovascular bundles and divide into medial and lateral branches after penetration of the muscular pelvis. The medial branches innervate smooth muscle component of the external urethral sphincter; the lateral branches continue to enter the cavernosal bodies

Separate authors have clearly shown several medial and lateral branches of the cavernosal nerves of the penis, although medial branches tend to accompany the urethra and lateral branches continue into the cavernosal bodies. The medial urethral branches might possibly participate in the smooth muscular innervation of the urethral sphincter. Destruction of these fibres during extended apical dissection of the prostate might jeopardise postoperative continence. As previously mentioned, the cavernosal nerves of the penis run in close proximity to the posterolateral aspects of the prostate. Beyond the apex of the prostate they run parallel to the urethra, traverse the muscular pelvis and breach the tunica albuginea to enter the cavernosal bodies (Fig. 2.1.4). Currently, there is heated debate concerning the communication with somatic branches of the pudendal nerve. However, cadaveric studies have clearly shown connections between the dorsal nerve and the cavernosal nerves of the penis at the level of the crura [21].

2.1.5 Pudendal Nerve

Ventral rami of spinal segments S2–4 form the pudendal nerve, which also receive parasympathetic and sympathetic fibres to form the pudendal plexus; therefore, it is accompanied by autonomic neural fibres. Sympathetic neural fibres run with the internal pudendal artery to the cavernosal bodies. The pudendal nerve emerges from the pudendal plexus as essentially a cutaneous nerve and exits the small pelvis together with the internal pudendal artery and vein. It runs in the direction of the ischial spine and emerges from the ischioanal fossa in a fascial sheath of the internal obturator muscle (Alcock's canal). At this point the nerve has left the levator "hammock". Division into the end branches – the perineal nerves and dorsal nerve of the penis – also occurs here. The deep branches of the perineal nerves (rami musculares) give motor supply to the striated urethral sphincter, ischiocavernosal muscles and bulbospongiosus muscle (Fig. 2.1.5). Superficial branches known as posterior scrotal rami supply the skin of the perineum and posterior scrotum. The rectal nerves innervate the external anal sphincter. The dorsal nerve of the penis

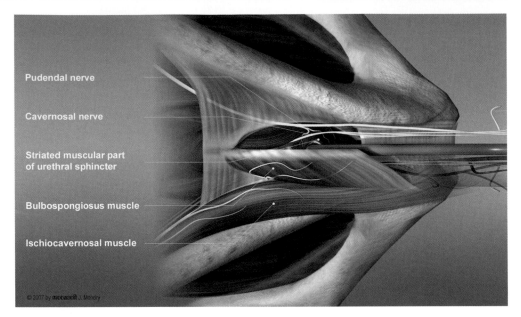

Fig. 2.1.5. The pudendal nerve gives off motor brances to the bulbospongiosus muscle, the ischiocavernosus muscle and the striated component of the external urethral sphincter

penetrates the suspensory ligament of the penis and supplies the penile shaft skin and glans penis.

Contraction of the bulbospongiosus and ischio-cavernosus muscles reduces venous drainage and leads to an intracavernosal pressure rise. Sensory afferences arise from the perineum and anal region as well as the posterior penile shaft and scrotum and undergo higher neural integration. In conclusion, the pudendal nerve is a somatosensory nerve with clear topographical separation from the cavernosal nerves of the penis, as shown in Fig. 2.1.5. Contrary to pelvic bone injuries and injuries related to vaginal delivery, intrapelvic operations involve negligible risk of injury to the pudendal nerve.

References

1. Stolzenburg JU, Rabenalt R, Tannapfel A, Liatsikos EN (2006) Intrafascial nerve-sparing endoscopic extraperitoneal radical prostatectomy. Urology 67:17–21
2. Walsh PC, Schlegel PN (1988) Radical pelvic surgery with preservation of sexual function. Ann Surg 208:391–400
3. Schlegel PN, Walsh PC (1987) Neuroanatomical approach to radical cystoprostatectomy with preservation of sexual function. J Urol 138:1402–1406
4. Leissner J, Allhoff EP, Wolff W, Feja C et al (2001) The pelvic plexus and antireflux surgery: topographical findings and clinical consequences. J Urol 165:1652–1655
5. Höckel M, Horn LC, Hentschel B, Höckel S et al (2003) Total mesometrial resection: high resolution nerve-sparing radical hysterectomy based on developmentally defined surgical anatomy. Int J Gynecol Cancer 13:791–803
6. Höckel M, Konerding MA, Heussel CP (1998) Liposuction-assisted nerve-sparing extended radical hysterectomy: oncologic rationale, surgical anatomy, and feasibility study. Am J Obstet Gynecol 178:971–976
7. Stelzner F, Fritsch H, Fleischhauer K (1989) The surgical anatomy of the genital nerves of the male and their preservation in excision of the rectum. Chirurg 60:228–234
8. Davis LP, Jelenko C (1975) Sexual function after abdominoperineal resection. South Med J 68:422–426
9. Lepor H, Gregerman M, Crosby R, Mostofi FK et al (1985) Precise localization of the autonomic nerves from the pelvic plexus to the corpora cavernosa: a detailed anatomical study of the adult male pelvis. J Urol 133:207–212
10. Menon M, Tewari A, Peabody J (2003) Vattikuti Institute prostatectomy: technique. J Urol 169:2289–2292
11. Costello AJ, Brooks M, Cole OJ (2004) Anatomical studies of the neurovascular bundle and cavernosal nerves. BJU Int 94:1071–1076
12. Kiyoshima K, Yokomizo A, Yoshida T, Tomita K et al (2004) Anatomical features of periprostatic tissue and its surroundings: a histological analysis of 79 radical retropubic prostatectomy specimens. Jpn J Clin Oncol 34:463–468

13. Eckhard C (1863) Untersuchungen über die Erection des Penis beim Hunde. Anat Physiol 3:123–166

14. Walsh PC, Donker PJ (1982) Impotence following radical prostatectomy: insight into etiology and prevention. J Urol 128:492–497

15. Müller J (1836) Über die organischen Nerven der erectilen männlichen Geschlechtsorgane des Menschen und der Säugetiere. Dümmler, Berlin

16. Budge JL (1858) Über das Centrum genitospinale. Virchows Arch p 15

17. Calabrisi P (1955) The nerve supply of the erectile cavernosus tissue of the genitalia in the human embryo and fetus. Department of Anatomy, George Washington University School of Medicine

18. Lue TF, Zeineh SJ, Schmidt RA, Tanagho EA (1984) Neuroanatomy of penile erection: its relevance to iatrogenic impotence. J Urol 131:273–280

19. Juenemann KP, Lue TF, Schmidt RA, Tanagho EA (1988) Clinical significance of sacral and pudendal nerve anatomy. J Urol 139:74–80

20. Fritsch H (1989) Topography of the pelvic autonomic nerves in human fetuses between 21–29 weeks of gestation. Anat Embryol (Berl) 180:57–64

21. Breza J, Aboseif SR, Orvis BR, Lue TF et al (1989) Detailed anatomy of penile neurovascular structures: surgical significance. J Urol 141:437–443

22. Stief CG, Djamilian M, Anton P, de RW et al (1991) Single potential analysis of cavernous electrical activity in impotent patients: a possible diagnostic method for autonomic cavernous dysfunction and cavernous smooth muscle degeneration. J Urol 146:771–776

23. Paick JS, Donatucci CF, Lue TF (1993) Anatomy of cavernous nerves distal to prostate: microdissection study in adult male cadavers. Urology 42:145–149

24. Zvara P, Carrier S, Kour NW, Tanagho EA (1994) The detailed neuroanatomy of the human striated urethral sphincter. Br J Urol 74:182–187

25. Strasser H, Klima G, Poisel S, Horninger W et al (1996) Anatomy and innervation of the rhabdosphincter of the male urethra. Prostate 28:24–31

26. Hoer J, Roegels A, Prescher A, Klosterhalfen B et al (2000) Preserving autonomic nerves in rectal surgery. Results of surgical preparation on human cadavers with fixed pelvic sections. Chirurg 71:1222–1229

27. Akita K, Sakamoto H, Sato T (2003) Origins and courses of the nervous branches to the male urethral sphincter. Surg Radiol Anat 25:387–392

28. Takenaka A, Kawada M, Murakami G, Hisasue S et al (2005) Interindividual variation in distribution of extramural ganglion cells in the male pelvis: a semi-quantitative and immunohistochemical study concerning nerve-sparing pelvic surgery. Eur Urol 48:46–52

Inter- and Intrafascial Dissection Technique of Nerve-Sparing Radical Prostatectomy

2.2

Jens-Uwe Stolzenburg · Jochen Neuhaus · Thilo Schwalenberg · Katharina Spanel-Borowski
Sabine Löffler · Rudolph Hohenfellner · Evangelos N. Liatsikos

The anatomy of the neurovascular bundle (NVB), the cavernosal nerves and the anatomic structures that surround the prostate have been evaluated in various studies [1–5]. Nevertheless, the nomenclature pertaining to the prostate's adjacent fascias and the level of dissection for a nerve-sparing procedure are under dispute.

Walsh describes the NVB as located between the two layers of the lateral pelvic fascia (levator fascia – lateral layer and prostatic fascia – medial layer). He states that during a nerve-sparing procedure, the prostatic fascia must remain on the prostate [3]. Menon et al. described their experience with robotic surgery at the Vattikuti Institute and suggested that the NVBs are enclosed within the layers of the periprostatic fascia, which is consisted of two thin layers that separate posteriorly in order to enclose the NVBs. The authors describe a triangular-shaped tunnel, formed from the two layers of the periprostatic fascia and the anterior layers of Denonvilliers' fascia, which is wide near the base and narrower near the apex. They state that while performing a nerve-sparing procedure, the periprostatic fascia must be incised anterior and parallel to the NVBs [1].

In 2004, Costello et al. showed that most of the NVB descends posterior to the seminal vesicle. The nerves converge to the mid-prostatic level but diverge once again as they approach the prostatic apex. The anterior and posterior nerves of the NVB are separated by about 3 cm at the level of the base of the prostate. At this anatomical point, the cavernosal nerves are not easily distinguished from the surrounding tissues and the surgeon must be careful during graft anastomosis to ensure the connection of all the nerve endings [4]. In the same year, Kiyoshima et al. proposed the wide dissection of the lateral aspect of the prostate during radical prostatectomy to ascertain NVB preservation. Although the NVB was thought to exist locally near the posterolateral region, it was found at the posterolateral region of the prostate in only 48% of the cases. In the remaining 52%, the nerves were spread over the entire lateral aspect of the prostate without either specific localisation or bundle formation. This typical distribution of nerve fibres around the prostate becomes clearly visible in a histological section from an embryo [6]. Moreover, Kiyoshima et al. described the lateral pelvic fascia as a multi-layered fascia, linked to the prostate capsule by collagen fibres. According to them, the site and the localisation of the NVB is related to the degree of fusion between prostate capsule and lateral pelvic fascia [2].

Since 1867, when Denonvilliers' fascia was illustrated in an anatomy text book, there has been continuing debate regarding the anatomy and embryological origins of all fascias [7]. Denonvilliers' fascia covers the prostate except for the ventral parts, the apex and the base and, cranially, the plexus vesicoprostaticus, the seminal vesicles and the ampullae of the ductus deferens. Laterally, it is interwoven with the fascia pelvis. Cranially, it merges into the subperitoneal connective tissue of the urinary bladder. Denonvilliers' fascia has been described to consist of a single layer, formed from fusion of two walls of the embryological peritoneal cul-de-sac [8]. Histologically, it has a double-layered quality which is not distinguishable intraoperatively. The fascia extends from the deepest point of the interprostatorectal peritoneal pouch to the pelvic floor and, contrary to the theory of Villers et al., does not lie forward of the anterior wall of the pouch. The posterior layer does not exist, and researchers who report such a layer are describing the rectal fascia propria [9].

We advocate the theory of one pelvic fascia covering the prostate and bladder, named "endopelvic fascia", finally inserting in the form of puboprostatic ligaments to the pubic bone. Furthermore, there is a connective tissue layer around the prostate ventrally

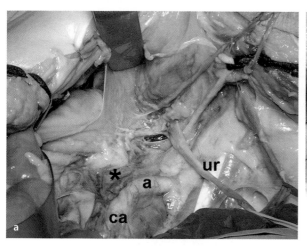
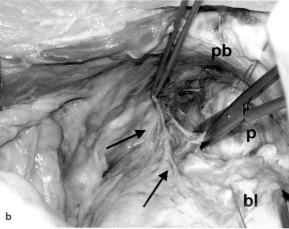
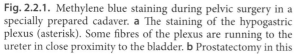

Fig. 2.2.1. Methylene blue staining during pelvic surgery in a specially prepared cadaver. **a** The staining of the hypogastric plexus (asterisk). Some fibres of the plexus are running to the ureter in close proximity to the bladder. **b** Prostatectomy in this cadaver (bladder neck and prostate are dissected), with abundant staining within the tissue (endopelvic fascia e.g.) lateral to the prostate

and laterally which can be named "periprostatic fascia". It is not clear whether such a fascia indeed exists, but there is certainly a plane of dissection between the prostate and its surrounding tissues. We have performed cadaveric studies and stained the fascias surrounding the prostate during a simulation of prostatectomy with methylene blue. Ehrlich was the first to describe the use of methylene blue to stain autonomic nerve fibres [10]. Seif et al. and Leissner et al. proposed the use of methylene blue staining for nerve-sparing operative procedures in urology [11, 12]. The technique of methylene blue staining in specially prepared cadavers (according to Thiel) has been used by Coers et al. to identify nerve fibres [13]. Figure 2.2.1a shows the staining of the hypogastric plexus in a stained cadaver. Figure 2.2.1b shows abundant staining within the endopelvic fascia. It has not been clearly demonstrated whether these lateral nerves are responsible for continence or erectile function. Nevertheless, the presence of nerves is clear and there is a tendency to maintain as many nerves as possible during a nerve-sparing procedure.

Takenada et al. advocate a trizonal anatomical concept. The tissue that they encountered during robotic radical prostatectomy was grouped in three broad zones, the proximal neurovascular plate, the predominant NVBs and the accessory distal neural pathways [15].

The terms extrafascial, interfascial and intrafascial are very often used to describe different dissection techniques, without clarifying the anatomical structures behind these terms. During non-nerve-sparing prostatectomy the endopelvic fascia is incised laterally close to the levator ani, allowing the "wide excision" of the prostate including its surrounding fascias and the NVBs. During intrafascial nerve-sparing endoscopic extraperitoneal prostatectomy (Fig. 2.2.2) we incise the endopelvic fascia only ventrally, medial to the puboprostatic ligaments. Then, we try to dissect on the prostatic capsule, freeing the prostate laterally from its thin surrounding fascia (periprostatic fascia) containing small vessels and nerves. The difference of our technique from the Vattikuti method is the preservation of all lateral enveloping periprostatic fascias. We only perform an anterior incision of the periprostatic fascia when carrying out an intrafascial nerve-sparing technique [16]. According to Kiyoshima et al. [2], this is a justified technical amendment in order to obtain integrity of the NVB.

The difference between the interfascial and intrafascial nerve-sparing radical prostatectomy techniques is shown in Fig. 2.2.3. In the interfascial technique, the endopelvic fascia is incised and the NVBs are spared posterolaterally between the endopelvic fascia and the periprostatic fascia (Fig. 2.2.3b). This technique is the standard nerve-sparing technique. That means that the periprostatic fascia remains on

2

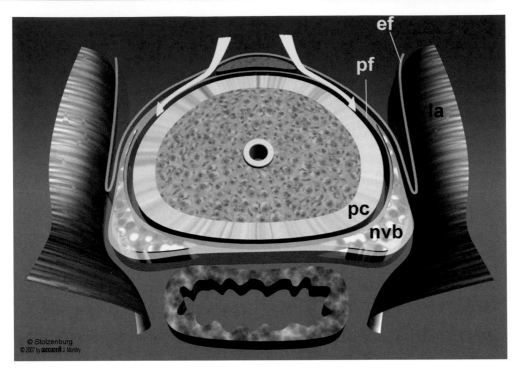

Fig. 2.2.2. Principles of intrafascial nerve-sparing radical prostatectomy. During the intrafascial nerve-sparing endoscopic extraperitoneal prostatectomy the endopelvic fascia is incised only ventrally medial to the puboprostatic ligaments. The dissection is performed on the prostatic capsule, freeing the prostate laterally from its thin surrounding fascia (periprostatic fascia) which contains small vessels and nerves. The dorsal dissection plane is between Denonvilliers' fascia and the prostatic capsule

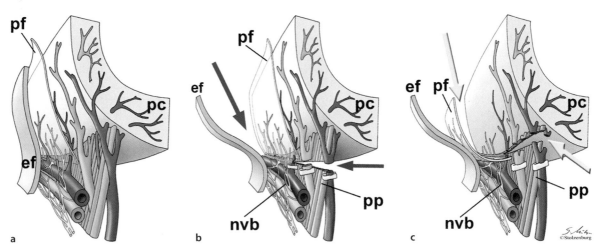

Fig. 2.2.3. Interfascial and intrafascial nerve-sparing radical prostatectomy. **a** The prostate is covered by endopelvic and periprostatic fascia. **b** In the interfascial technique, the endopelvic fascia is incised and the neurovascular bundles are spared posterolaterally. **c** In the intrafascial technique, the endopelvic fascia, the periprostatic fascia and Denonvilliers' fascia are not a part of the specimen because the dissection plane is directly on the prostatic capsule

the prostate. In the intrafascial technique, the endopelvic fascia, the periprostatic fascia and Denonvilliers' fascia are not a part of the specimen (Fig. 3c) because the dissection plane is directly on the prostatic capsule.

References

1. Menon M, Tewari A, Peabody J et al (2003) Vattikuti Institute prostatectomy: technique. J Urol 169:2289–2292
2. Kiyoshima K, Yokomizo A, Yoshida T, Tomita K, Yonemasu H, Nakamura M, Oda Y, Naito S, Hasegawa Y (2004) Anatomical features of periprostatic tissue and its surroundings: a histological analysis of 79 radical retropubic prostatectomy specimens. Jpn J Clin Oncol 34:463–468
3. Walsh PC (1998) Anatomic radical prostatectomy: evolution of the surgical technique. J Urol 160:2418–2424
4. Costello AJ, Brooks M, Cole OJ (2004) Anatomical studies of the neurovascular bundle and cavernosal nerves. BJU Int 94:1071–1076
5. McCarthy JF, Catalona WJ (1996) Nerve sparing radical retropubic prostatectomy. In: Marshall FF (ed): Textbook of operative urology. Saunders, Philadelphia, pp 537–544
6. Stolzenburg JU, Schwalenberg T, Horn LC, Neuhaus J, Constantinides C, Liatsikos EN (2006) Anatomical hazards of radical prostatecomy. Eur Urol 51:629–639
7. Dietrich H (1997) Giovanni Domenico Santorini (1681–1737). Charles-Pierre Denonvilliers (1808–1872). First description of urosurgically relevant structures in the small pelvis. Eur Urol 32:124–127
8. Van Ophonen A, Roth S (1997) The anatomy and embryological origins of the fascia of Denonvilliers: A medico-historical debate. J Urol 157:3–9
9. Villers A, Mcneal JE, Freiha FS, Boccon-Gibod L, Stamey TA (1993) Invasion of Denonvilliers' fascia in radical prostatectomy specimens. J Urol 149:793
10. Ehrlich P (1885) Zur biologischen Verwertung des Methylenblau. Zbl Med Wiss 23:113–117
11. Seif C, Martinez Portillo FJ, Osmonov DK, Bohler G, van der Horst C, Leissner J,Hohenfellner R, Juenemann KP, Braun PM (2004) Methylene blue staining for nerve-sparing operative procedures: an animal model. Urology 63:1205–1208
12. Leissner J,Allhoff EP, Wolff W, Feja C, Hockel M, Black P, Hohenfellner R (2001) The pelvic plexus and antireflux surgery: topographical findings and clinical consequences. J Urol 165:1652–1655
13. Coers CD, Woolf AL (1959) The innervation of muscle: a biopsy study. Oxford, Blackwell
14. Takenaka A, Leung RA, Fujisawa M, Tewari AK (2006) Anatomy of autonomic nerve component in the male pelvis: the new concept from a perspective for robotic nerve-sparing radical prostatectomy. World J Urol 24:136–143
15. Stolzenburg JU, Rabenalt R, Tannapfel A, Liatsikos EN (2006) Intrafascial nerve-sparing endoscopic extraperitoneal radical prostatectomy. Urology. 67:17–21

Jens-Uwe Stolzenburg · Jochen Neuhaus · Lars-Christian Horn · Evangelos N. Liatsikos · Thilo Schwalenberg

The external sphincter (urethral sphincter) ensures continence after radical prostatectomy. The main goal of the surgeon should be the protection of the urethral sphincter, even though the internal sphincter (vesical sphincter) and the pelvic floor muscles also contribute to the continence mechanism. There is controversy in the literature regarding the course and structure of the urethral sphincter. Most important for prostate surgery is the apex of the prostate, as at this level striated muscle fibres of the external urethral sphincter are already prominent at the ventral aspect. Furthermore, at the apex of the prostate there is the most intimate contact between the external sphincter, the puboprostatic ligaments and the endopelvic fascia. It is generally accepted that the urethral sphincter is a distinct muscular structure and is not part of the pelvic floor musculature (even though they are adjacent structures). There is no muscular connection to the levator ani muscle [1–3].

We have performed a study to clarify the structure of the muscular systems of the lower urinary tract, from the bulb of the penis up to the actual bladder neck. Fifty autopsy preparations from males of all ages, from newborn to 82 years, were examined. In order to preserve their anatomical interrelationships, all organs of the lower urinary tract (urinary bladder, bladder neck, urethra) and surrounding organs (pros-

tate, seminal vesicles, symphysis, rectum, musculature of the pelvic floor) were anatomically dissected and fixed in buffered 4% formalin. In so doing, all tissue around the urethra was preserved. The fixed organ blocks were completely cut on a modified microtome (Tetrander Jung) in serial sections at a thickness of 10 μm. Serial sections were made in frontal (coronal), sagittal and transverse (horizontal) planes and were stained with resorcin–fuchsin, haematoxylin–eosin, Crossmon trichrome staining, silver stain and by smooth muscle cell α-actin immunohistochemistry. All serial sections were systematically examined at different magnifications [1]. Figure 2.3.1 shows histological images from a transverse section series from a newborn. It is evident that the external sphincter is a separate musculature with a boundary layer of connective tissue separating it from the surrounding pelvic musculature. Histomorphological investigations and magnetic resonance imaging in adults have confirmed this morphological fact [4–6]. In many textbooks a transversus perinei profundus muscle is described as part of the "urogenital diaphragm". As is shown in Fig. 2.3.1 and has been documented in our published study [4], we were not able to confirm the existence of this muscle structure. Thus we consider the urethral sphincter to be an autonomous muscular unit in all age groups.

Fig. 2.3.1. Transverse sections of a male newborn (Crossmon staining). The series starts at the level of the verumontanum (**a**) and ends at the bulbus penis, depicting the bulbourethral glands (**d**). The external sphincter is a separate musculature with a boundary layer of connective tissue (*arrows*) in the alignment towards the surrounding pelvic musculature. *us*, Urethral sphincter; *p*, prostate; *sy*, symphysis; *oi*, obturator internus; *oe*, obturator externus; *la*, levator ani; *bg*, bulbourethralis glands (Cowper's glands); *ul*, urethral lumen

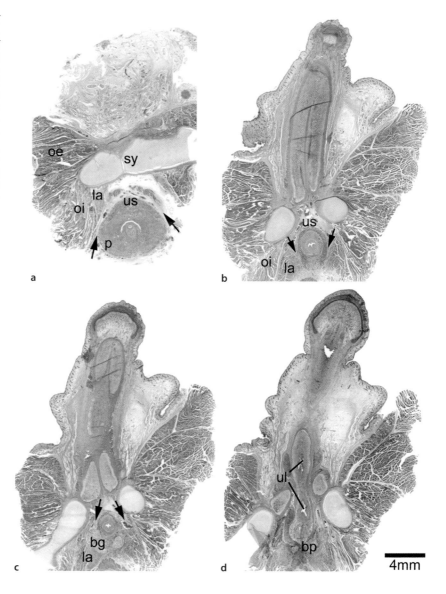

2.3.1 Components of the Urethral Sphincter

The urethral sphincter is horseshoe shaped and does not converge dorsally, where muscular fibres insert in a strongly built "raphe" of connective tissue which again serves as an anchor for the external sphincter in the boundary layer towards the rectum. Some groups prefer the description "omega shaped" rather than "horseshoe shaped" [5–8]. Although the shape seems to be broadly accepted, there is no concurrence re-

garding the course and structure of the urethral sphincter. Dorschner et al. were the first to describe two parts of the urethral sphincter – the outer striated and the inner smooth muscular component – both of them horseshoe shaped. Dorschner and Stolzenburg first reported the terms musculus sphincter urethrae glaber (smooth muscular part of the urethral sphincter) and musculus sphincter urethrae transversostriatus (striated part of the urethral sphincter) [9]. Strasser et al. have referred to the external urethral

2

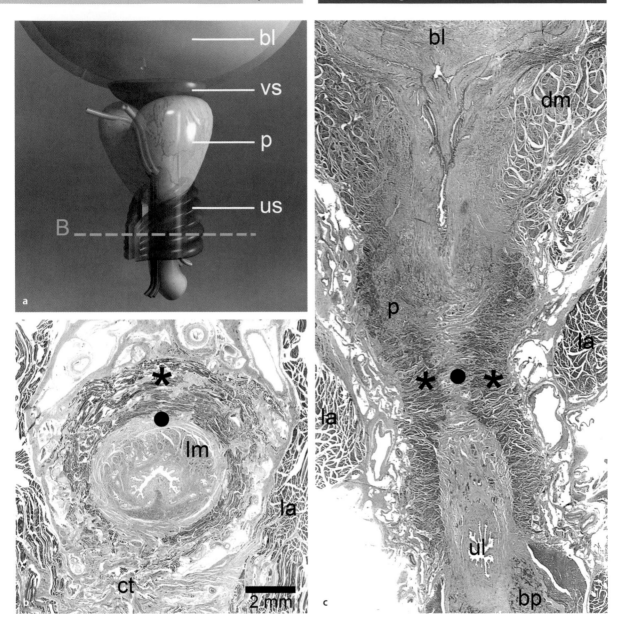

Fig. 2.3.2. a Three-dimensional model of the male lower urinary tract. **b** Transverse section through the external urethral sphincter system of a 56-year-old male. **c** Frontal section of a 7 year old male. Muscle tissue is *red* and connective tissue is *blue–green* in the histological sections (Crossmon staining). The external urethral sphincter is composed of a strongly developed striated part (*star*) and a thinner smooth muscular part (*dot*). There is no muscular connection to the pelvic floor musculature. *bl*, Bladder; *vs*, vesical sphincter; *p*, prostate; *us*, urethral sphincter (striated part); *dm*, detrusor muscle; *la*, levator ani; *lm*, longitudinal muscle system; *ct*, connective tissue; *ul*, urethral lumen; *bp*, bulb of penis; *star*, striated; *dot*, smooth

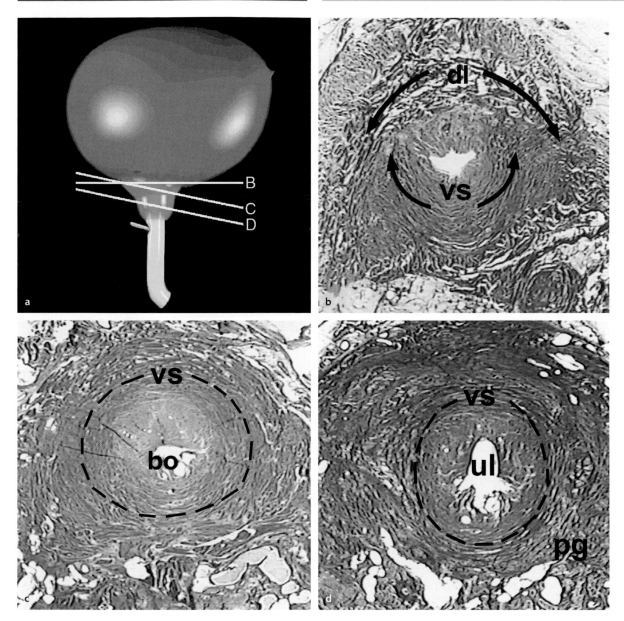

Fig. 2.3.3. a Model of the male lower urinary tract without the prostate. The internal vesical sphincter is shown in *green*. The different planes of the histological sections are indicated (*b–d*). The "wrong" section plane **b** gives the impression of two distinct muscular structures forming a loop system around the bladder neck, whereas section planes **c** and **d** clearly demonstrate a ring-shaped unique internal (vesical) sphincter. *dl*, Detrusor lamellae; *vs*, vesical sphincter; *bo*, bladder outlet; *pg*, prostate glands; *ul*, urethral lumen

sphincter as a rhabdosphincter. This term suggests that the external sphincter is an exclusively striated muscle [3, 7].

From histomorphological investigations it is clear that there is a smooth muscular sheet (dot in Fig. 2.3.2) under the external striated muscle layer (star in Fig. 2.3.2). This smooth muscular part of the external sphincter is likely to ensure continence at rest after resection of the internal vesical sphincter during radical prostatectomy or transurethral resection. Histological and functional observations support the notion that the smooth muscular part of the external urethral sphincter is mainly responsible for continence at rest while the striated part provides reflex continence during stress [9].

Several authors promote the notion that continence at rest is also mediated by the striated urethral sphincter. Indeed, some studies have demonstrated that the striated external sphincter is made up of two different striated muscle fibre types, the slow and the fast twitch fibres [10]. The 'fast twitch' fibres are thought to compensate for sudden abdominal pressure increases. In males the proportion of 'fast twitch fibres' is 65%, whilst in females it is 13%. The 'slow twitch fibres' contribute to sustained urethral pressure during filling [11]. In an effort to explain postoperative urine continence, investigators hypothesised that under certain conditions (i.e. in the absence of smooth muscular vesical sphincter), the fibre type becomes interchangeable. The switch to slow twitch fibres should ensure continuous continence. Some have postulated a threefold innervation of the striated urethral musculature by somatic, sympathetic and parasympathetic nerve fibres [12]. Nevertheless, the concept of triple innervation of the urethral sphincter must be viewed with caution.

During radical prostatectomy attention in surgical dissection of the sphincter is focused on the integrity of the urethral sphincter. Bladder neck-sparing prostatectomy also involves the vesical sphincter, which continues to be a subject of heated debate in the literature.

2.3.2 Vesical Sphincter

Former assumptions that the vesical sphincter could be formed out of muscular slings from the detrusor are contrary to current opinion. There is overall agreement on the existence of a distinct muscular structure but no consensus on the composition of the

muscle. Some authors regard the continuation of the detrusor lamellae to be the origin of all urethral musculature [13, 14]. Others favour the concept of a floor panel when describing the vesical sphincter [15, 16]. This panel is thought to consist ventrally of the detrusor muscle und dorsally of trigonal musculature. In our own study we showed that in a strictly transverse dissection this structure really appears to be composed of two different muscles (Fig. 2.3.3b), but the bladder neck is not positioned in a totally perpendicular plane. The physiological position of the entire bladder neck has an oblique direction. Changing the histological investigation plane accordingly, we were able to identify a distinct muscle surrounding in a circular manner the bladder neck, which is called internal or vesical sphincter (musculus sphincter vesicae) [17]. Lamellae of the detrusor do not participate in the formation of this muscle (Fig. 2.3.3c, d).

2.3.3 Urethral Muscles and Radical Prostatectomy

A further point of controversy is the craniocaudal extension of the external sphincter over the prostate and bladder. Dorschner's groups and others advocate that the urethral sphincter is ventrally more strongly developed. Furthermore, the apex of the prostate is ventrally overlapped by the striated muscle fibres of the external urethral sphincter. In contrast, Oelrich et al. and Myers et al. described a vertically orientated sphincter muscle system, from the base of the bladder to the bulb of the penis [18, 19]. Interestingly, Dorschner et al. found two vertically orientated muscles in the urethral muscular sheet, the ventrolateral longitudinal muscle and the dorsal longitudinal muscle (2.3.4) [20–22]. The interpretation of the various longitudinally orientated muscular structures remains unclear.

During radical prostatectomy we are able to identify and preserve three muscular structures. The ring-shaped vesical (internal) sphincter can be preserved during bladder neck-sparing radical prostatectomy. However, this is not always possible due to anatomic variation in the shape of the prostate (e.g. large middle lobe). The most important component responsible for postoperative urinary continence is the circularly orientated, horseshoe-shaped urethral sphincter. The main difficulty for the surgeon is the inability to identify intraoperatively the exact border of the projection of the urethral sphincter, overlapping approximately

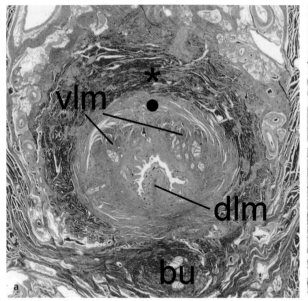
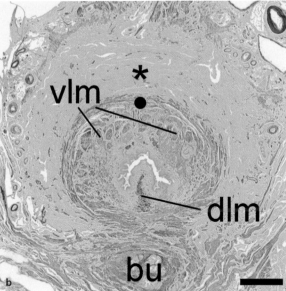

Fig. 2.3.4. Transversal adjacent sections of an adult male distal urethra. **a** Crossmon staining; **b** smooth muscle cell α-actin immunolabelling. The two parts (*star*, striated; *dot*, smooth) of the horseshoe-shaped external sphincter are clearly evident. In **b** the striated part is not stained. Furthermore, longitudinal muscle cell bundles can be shown. The ventrolateral longitudinal muscle (*vlm*) consists of large muscle cell bundles separated by perimysial connective tissue and urethral glands. The dorsal longitudinal muscle (*dlm*) is composed of small, closely arranged smooth muscle cell bundles. *Scale bar* 10 mm

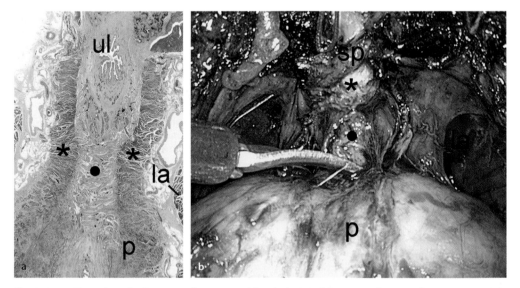

Fig. 2.3.5. a Frontal urethral section of a 17-year-old male. **b** Apical dissection during endoscopic extraperitoneal radical prostatectomy demonstrating the three steps of this procedure:. step 1, Santorini plexus (*sp*); step 2, junction between urethral sphincter and apex (*star*); step 3: inner smooth muscular layer (*dot*). *ul*, Urethral lumen; *la*, levator ani muscle; *p*, prostate; *sp*, Santorini plexus

2

one third of the prostate. Thus, many surgeons start apical dissection proximally on the prostatic surface as a mixture of blunt and sharp dissection. Nevertheless, this remains an unclear field that merits further investigation.

The third component of the muscular complex that can be preserved during radical prostatectomy is the vertically (longitudinally) oriented smooth muscle component of the urethral musculature. This inner muscular layer (close to the urethral lumen) can be identified and dissected (Fig. 2.3.5b). Surgeons performing perineal prostatectomy dissect this layer as long as possible. Laparoscopists and surgeons performing open radical retropubic prostatectomy attempt the same by retracting the prostate during apical dissection to gain maximum urethral length. Nevertheless, it is still unclear whether the technique of maintaining a long inner smooth muscular urethral component has any effect on postoperative urinary continence. We always try to keep this part of the urethra as long as possible.

Summarising, we suggest that apical dissection should be performed as a three-step procedure. The Santorini plexus and the overlying connective and areolar tissue are initially dissected, followed by dissection of the junction between the urethral sphincter (star in Fig. 2.3.5) and the apex. Finally, the inner smooth muscular layer (dot in Fig. 2.3.5) of the urethra is freed and dissected.

References

1. Dorschner W, Stolzenburg JU, Neuhaus J (2001) Structure and function of the bladder neck. In: Advances in anatomy, embryology and cell biology. Springer, Berlin Heidelberg New York, pp 31–39
2. Kaye KW, Milne N, Creed K, van der Werf B (1997) The 'urogenital diaphragm', external urethral sphincter and radical prostatectomy. 1. Aust N Z J Surg 67:40–44
3. Strasser H, Bartsch G (2000) Anatomy and innervation of the rhabdosphincter of the male urethra. Semin Urol Oncol 18:2–8
4. Dorschner W, Biesold M, Schmidt F, Stolzenburg JU (1999) The dispute about the external sphincter and the urogenital diaphragm. J Urol 162:1942–1945
5. Sebe P, Schwentner C, Oswald J, Radmayr C, Bartsch G, Fritsch H (2005) Fetal development of striated and smooth muscle sphincters of the male urethra from a common primordium and modifications due to the development of the prostate: an anatomic and histologic study. Prostate 62:388–393
6. Fritsch H, Lienemann A, Brenner E, Ludikowski B (2004) Clinical anatomy of the pelvic floor. Adv Anat Embryol Cell Biol 175:III-IX, 1–64
7. Strasser H, Klima G, Poisel S, Horninger W, Bartsch G (1996) Anatomy and innervation of the rhabdosphincter of the male urethra. Prostate 28:24–31
8. Ludwikowski B, Oesch Hayward I, Brenner E, Fritsch H (2001) The development of the external urethral sphincter in humans. BJU Int 87:565–568
9. Dorschner W, Stolzenburg JU (1994) A new theory of micturition and urinary continence based on histomorphological studies. 3. The two parts of the Musculus sphincter urethrae: physiological importance for continence in rest and stress. Urol Int 52:185–188
10. Schroder HD, Reske-Nielsen E (1983) Fiber types in the striated urethral and anal sphincters. Acta Neuropathol (Berl) 60:278–282
11. Brading AF (1999) The physiology of the mammalian urinary outflow tract. Exp Physiol 84:215–121
12. Elbadawi A, Schenk EA (1974) A new theory of the innervation of bladder musculature. 2. Innervation of the vesicourethral junction and external urethral sphincter. J Urol 111:613–615
13. Lapides J (1958) Structure and function of internal sphincter. J Urol 80:341–353
14. Tanagho EA (1973) Vesicourethral dynamics. In: Lutzeyer W, Melchior H (eds) Urodynamics. Springer, Berlin Heidelberg New York, p 215
15. Hutch JA, Shopfner CE (1968) A new theory of the anatomy of the anatomy of the internal urinary sphincter and the physiology of micturation. The base plate and enuresis. J Urol 99:174–177
16. Hutch JA (1971) The internal urinary sphincter: A double loop system. J Urol 105:375–383
17. Dorschner W, Stolzenburg JU, Dietrich F (1994) A new theory of micturation and urinary continence based on histomorphological studies. 2. The musculus sphincter vesicae: continence or sexual function? Urol Int 52:154–158
18. Oelrich TM (1980) The urethral sphincter muscle in the male. Am J Anat 158:229–246
19. Myers RP, Goellner JR, Cahill DR (1987) Prostate shape, external striated urethral sphincter and radical prostatectomy: the apical dissection. J Urol 138: 543–550
20. Dorschner W, Rothe P, Leutert G (1989) Die urethrale Längsmuskulatur. Verh Anat Ges 82:801–803
21. Dorschner W, Stolzenburg JU, Rassler J (1994) A new theory of micturition and urinary continence based on histomorphological studies. 4. The musculus dilatator urethrae: force of micturition. Urol Int 52:189–193
22. Dorschner W, Stolzenburg JU (1994) A new theory of micturation and urinary continence based on histomorphological studies. 5. The musculus ejaculatorius: a newly described structure responsible for seminal emission and ejaculation. Urol Int 53:34–37

Equipment for EERPE

3

Contents

Jens-Uwe Stolzenburg

HD EndoEYE

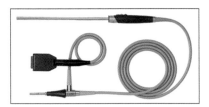

	Instrument name	Qty
WA50010A	Video telescope "HD EndoEYE", 0° direction of view, 10 mm, 325 mm working length, autoclavable	1

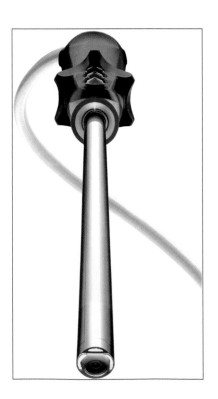

- **High Definition (HDTV) Video Chip – for a Revolutionary Image**
  The HD EndoEYE video laparoscope in combination with the EVIS EXERA II system sets a new benchmark of excellence for laparoscopic imaging with the introduction of HDTV to the O.R.
  By placing the high definition video chip at the distal tip of the scope, the image is sensed, transmitted and processed directly without interfering interfaces.

- **All-in-One – for Outstanding Ease of Use**
  HD EndoEYE does not require assembling – just plug and play!
  Gone are the days of adjusting the camera head and connecting the light-guide cable. There is no possibility of fogging or a loose connection to the camera head.

Ultrasonic Surgical System

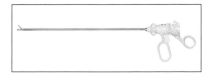

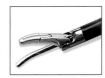

	Instrument name	Qty
N2301560	SonoSurg scissors "T3105", 5 mm, long, HF connector, curved tip	1
alternatively		
N2301460	SonoSurg scissors "T3100", 5 mm, long, HF connector, straight tip	1
A90222A	Wrench "MAJ-1117", torque, for 5 mm instruments	1
A90205A	Transducer "SonoSurg-T2H", for 5 mm probes	1

Suction and Irrigation System

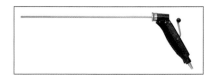

	Instrument name	Qty
WA51172L	Handle set, "HiQ+" suction/irrigation, 8 mm	1
	Suction/irrigation tube, distal holes,	
WA51131A	5.3 x 360 mm	1
WA51151A	10 x 360 mm	1

Suture Material

	Instrument name	Qty
	(To fix Hasson trocar) Vicryl TN 2/0	2
	(Santorini Plexus)	
CL883	Polysorb GS 22 2/0, 75 cm	1
alternatively	Vicryl SH 2/0	1
	(Anastomosis)	
UL878	Polysorb GU-46 2/0, 75 cm	4
alternatively	Vicry UR 6 2/0	4
	(Intracutaneous skin suture)	
SC5618G	Caprosyn P-12 3/0, 45 cm	2

3

Hand Instruments

	Instrument name	Qty
WA63708A WA63718A	Needle holder "HiQ+", 5 x 330 mm, with ratchet, straight curved 1	1
A63010A	Grasping forceps "HiQ+", atraumatic, with Ergo handle, 5 x 330 mm, with ratchet	2
A63310A A63320A	Dissection forceps "HiQ+", with Ergo handle, 5 x 330 mm, straight 5 x 330 mm, Maryland	2 1
A63810A	Scissors "HiQ+", Metzenbaum, with Ergo handle, 5 x 330 mm	1
A56790A	Clip applicator, 10 x 330 mm, curved, for clips medium/large A5635	1

Bipolar Forceps

	Instrument name	Qty
WA63120C	Grasping forceps "HiQ+", Johann, fenestrated, with Ergo handle, 5 x 330 mm, bipolar	1
A60003C	HF cable, bipolar, 3.5 m length, for UES-30/-40, and Valleylab HF units	1

Trocars

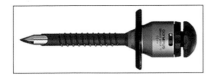

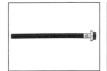

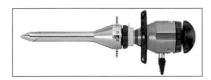

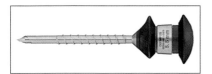

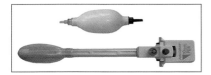

	Instrument name	Qty
A5859	Trocar "TroQ", 11 x 80 mm, Trocar tube, with thread and stopcock	1
A5823	Trocar spike, triangular tip	1
	Reduction tube,	
A5610	10 mm to 5 mm, insulated	1
A5837	13/11 mm to 5 mm	1
	Trocar "TroQ", 11 x 110 mm,	
A5828	Trocar tube, with stopcock	1
A5855	Trocar spike, according to Hasson	1
A5887	Trocar cone, for trocar acc. to Hasson	1
	Trocar "TroQ^{SL}", 5.5 x 80 mm,	
A5819	Trocar tube, with thread	3
A5948	Trocar spike, triangular	3
OMSPDB 1000	Tyco Balloon Trocar PDB 1000	1

Accessories

	Instrument name	Qty
ECatch10G	Tyco retrieval bag "EndoCatch"	1
	18 Fr. catheter	1
	18 Fr. silicon (final) catheter	1
	Bladder syringe	1
	Langenbeck Retractors, 43 x 13 mm	2

The Tower

3

Components/Devices

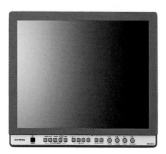

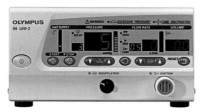

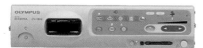

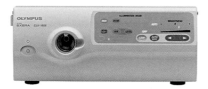

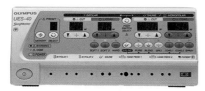

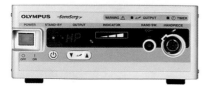

Olympus peripheral equipment for advanced endoscopic procedures:

Monitor – OEV191H
Full digital HDTV high-resolution images with stable, flicker-free image quality

Insufflator – UHI-3
The UHI-3 allows you to keep your full concentration where it belongs. Its smoke evacuation maintains clear operative views, while the 35 l/min insufflation quickly responds to gas leaks.

EVIS EXERA II Video System Center CV-180
EXERA II is the first video platform introducing 1080i HDTV to all fields of endoscopic imaging.

Light Source – CLV-180
The high-quality 300 W xenon lamp provides illumination ideal for endoscopy, allowing observation in deep sites or advanced techniques with standard and high intensity mode.

HF Unit – UES-40
The Olympus UES-40 SurgMaster – one generator for virtually any electrosurgical need

Ultrasonic Surgical System – SonoSurg G2
The versatile, safe and amazingly efficient SonoSurg from Olympus offers an outstanding cost performance thanks to fully autoclavable, reusable parts.

Advances in Image Processing

Thorsten Lüdtke · Christine Senet

Improvement in image processing is one of the factors that helps us to perform more complex procedures than some years ago while further broadening the applications of laparoscopy. „A better video image may result in better endoscopic surgery" is not a new notion [1]. With exceptional imaging quality, minimally invasive surgery will reach new levels of precision and reliability [2].

Minimally invasive surgery strongly depends on imaging [3]. Consequently, higher resolution yielding more detailed information is of great concern for surgeons. The availability of high-definition television (HDTV) for surgical endoscopy offers the surgeon more information to work within the three-dimensions increasing the sense of realism. Having HDTV image quality on screen during minimally invasive surgery might lead to increased accuracy, fewer errors and less surgeon fatigue.

Another innovation in the field of minimally invasive surgery is narrow-band imaging (NBI). NBI visualises fine capillary patterns and vessel networks underneath the mucosal surface, in addition to conventional white-light observation [4]. NBI is based on wavelength-selective absorption and scattering of light in tissue layers. By a selection of certain wavelength bandwidths it is possible to limit the depth of the observed tissue layer. The evaluation of this brand-new technology in the surgical field has so far shown a potential for applications such as sigmoidectomy, and it may also be applicable for better visualisation of carcinoma in situ in the bladder.

For years surgeons have been discussing how to combine minimal invasive surgical interventions with intraluminal imaging, e.g. for colorectal or bariatric surgery as well as for cystectomy, and the potential medical benefits that would arise. Accordingly, it is important that the latest imaging platforms are compatible for surgical and endoscopic applications.

3.2.1 High-Resolution Images

In surgical endoscopy HDTV is not simply a question of displaying crystal-clear images with natural colour, but also a question of developing an imaging chain that is 100% HDTV compatible from the scope's CCD chip to the monitor.

HDTV images are composed of almost double the number of scanning lines (1080 vs. 576) used in conventional video systems. This higher number of scanning lines yields a marked increase in image information and produces a picture that is sharp and detailed, with accurate rendition of even minute capillaries and subtle mucosal structures throughout the area shown on the screen.

3.2.2 What Is HDTV?

HDTV is a term for broadcasting standards with higher resolution than traditional formats. Two HDTV standards are now adopted as global standards: vertical resolution of 1080 active lines or 720 active lines.

3.2.3 Highlighting Hidden Tissue Structures with NBI

Narrow-band imaging (NBI) capability enhances the visibility of capillaries and other minuscule structures on the mucosal surface. Due to the biological characteristics of tissue, narrow-band light is absorbed and scattered differently in the mucosa compared to white light with a wider spectrum. This emphasises the contrast between small vessels and normal tissue as well as minute structures within the upper mucosa layers. The newest systems available feature dedicated optical light-filtering technology and provide considerable advantages over digital filtering methods. The improved visibility made possible by NBI may prove to be as good as chromoendoscopy but much easier to handle [5]. Another advantage of new imaging systems in comparison to chromoendoscopy is that it allows surgeons to switch between regular and NBI images during the procedure as often as necessary.

In the upper gastrointestinal tract, NBI helps to identify areas of intestinal metaplasia within columnar mucosa in the distal oesophagus. It can also identify specific patterns associated with Barrett's oesophagus, which may represent lesions of high-grade dysplasia. In the lower gastrointestinal tract, NBI emphasises pit patterns as well as chromoendoscopy in the colon. In addition to helping improve detection of lesions in the colon, NBI helps identify suspicious areas for target biopsies in patients with ulcerative colitis. After these first applications in gastrointestinal diagnosis and therapeutic procedures, NBI has recently been discussed for use in detection of carcinoma in situ of the bladder.

References

1. van Bergen P, Kunert W, Buess GF (2000) The effect of high-definition imaging on surgical task efficiency in minimally invasive surgery: an experimental comparison between three-dimensional imaging and direct vision through a stereoscopic TEM rectoscope.. Surg Endosc 14:71–74
2. Tan YH, Preminger GM (2004) Advances in video and imaging in ureteroscopy.. Urol Clin North Am 31:33–42
3. Way LW, Stewart L, Gantert W, Liu K, Lee CM, Whang K, Hunter JG (2003) Causes and prevention of laparoscopic bile duct injuries: analysis of 252 cases from a human factors and cognitive psychology perspective. Ann Surg 237:460–469
4. Kuznetsov K, Lambert R, Rey JF (2006) Narrow-band imaging: potential and limitations. Endoscopy 38:76–81
5. Kara MA, Peters FP, Rosmolen WD, Krishnadath KK, ten Kate FJ, Fockens P, Bergman JJ (2005) High-resolution endoscopy plus chromoendoscopy or narrow-band imaging in Barrett's esophagus: a prospective randomized crossover study.. Endoscopy 37:929–936

Indications for Endoscopic Extraperitoneal Radical Prostatectomy

4

Jens-Uwe Stolzenburg · Evangelos Liatsikos · Lars-Christian Horn · Michael C. Truss

Contents

4

The indications for endoscopic extraperitoneal radical prostatectomy (EERPE) are the same as for open radical retropubic prostatectomy. Clinically localized prostate cancer (T1 and T2) is the most important indication for treatment. The life expectancy of the patients should be at least 10 years. There are no specific selection criteria or special contraindications for EERPE.

There is a continuous debate in the literature regarding the operative management of T3 carcinoma of the prostate. Only few published studies report on the treatment outcomes in patients with clinical T3 disease. Surgical treatment of clinical stage T3 carcinoma is debatable and for some authors even contraindicated, mainly due to an increased risk of positive surgical margins, lymph node metastases, and a less favorable long-term outcome. Nevertheless, there are no randomized clinical trials comparing treatment options and their respective long-term outcomes in such patients. Various authors report that 15–25% of all clinical stage T3 tumors were overstaged (cT3, pT2), while only 8% were understaged (cT3, pT4). Overstaged patients tend to have a favorable prognosis, while most pT3b patients developed early disease progression [1].

According to the 2006 EAU guidelines on prostate cancer the overall PSA-free survival rate is approximately 20% after 5 years for clinical T3 cancer patients [1]. Tumor Gleason score has a clear impact on long-term outcome, even though biopsy and specimen findings often do not concur. Several authors advocate that radical prostatectomy for clinical T3a cancer with a PSA <10 ng/ml can reach a 5-year PSA-free survival rate of approximately 60% (European Association of Urology Guidelines, 2006 edition).

In contrast, in one large recent study from a single center, improved medium-term outcomes (19% PSA recurrence rate) were reported in patients with positive surgical margins after a mean follow-up of 45.8 months [2]. These excellent data may fuel the discussion on the role of surgery in cT3 prostate cancer in the future.

Further arguments in favor of surgical treatment for clinical T3 tumors are the possibility of adjuvant external beam radiotherapy (e.g. intensity-modulated radiotherapy) in the case of positive margins, and the avoidance of local complications (e.g. hematuria, retention due to clot formation, ureteral obstruction).

According to the European Association of Urology Guidelines (2006 edition), surgery can be considered as a therapeutic alternative for patients with clinical T3a carcinoma of the prostate. Both patients with clinically overstaged tumors (pT2) and those with pT3a tumors can benefit from surgical treatment [1].

Laparoscopic/endoscopic radical prostatectomy for clinical T3 cancer for the prostate requires extensive surgical experience and should be avoided by beginners.

4.1 Nerve-sparing EERPE

Preservation of normal erectile function is possible in selected patients by unilateral or bilateral preservation of the neurovascular bundles. For appropriate stage evaluation of the tumor, standard biopsy with at least 12 samples is mandatory. Criteria for the performance of a nerve-sparing technique are the following:

1. Preoperative erectile function sufficient for intercourse. This is a relative indication, since also the return to complete continence seems to be better following a nerve-sparing procedure. Therefore, a nerve-sparing procedure may also be indicated in patients with impaired sexual function [3].
2. Clinically organ-confined prostate cancer.
3. No palpable induration at the apex or posterolateral margins of the prostate. In selected cases intraoperative frozen section may be helpful to decide whether or not a nerve-sparing technique should be performed.
4. Patients with PSA <10 ng/ml and Gleason score <7 traditionally are regarded as candidates for a nerve-sparing procedure; however, those with a less favorable profile may also be considered on an individual basis. As in patients with a palpable lesion or a Gleason score of 7, intraoperative frozen section may be helpful in this setting. Newer normograms taking into account the percentage of tumor infiltration per biopsy, total number of biopsies and number of positive biopsies may aid decision making in the future.

Contraindications for the performance of a nerve-sparing technique are the following:
1. Prostate cancer with a Gleason score of 8–10. In the case of unilateral Gleason 8 disease, then a nerve-sparing procedure can be performed contralaterally by an experienced surgeon.

2. Fixation of the neurovascular bundle to the prostatic capsule (intraoperative decision).
3. Tumor invasion within the neurovascular bundle (intraoperative frozen section).
4. Induration at the apex or posterolateral borders of the prostate.

4.2 Contraindications for EERPE

There are no specific contraindications for EERPE. Patients suitable for surgery are also candidates for EERPE. Contraindications for surgery in general are:
- Serious cardiac conditions (intracardiac shunts, severe aortic or mitral valve insufficiency); severe cardiac insufficiency (NYHA III–IV); high intracranial and intraocular pressure (risk of intracranial or retinal hemorrhage)
- Uncorrected coagulopathy

4.3 Preoperative Preparation

We administer an enema on the evening before surgery and one early in the morning of the operative day. No further bowel preparation is necessary. Additional epidural anesthesia is not required.

The risk of requiring blood transfusion in our experience is under 1%. Therefore the patients are not advised to donate autologous blood. Broad-spectrum antibiotics are administered perioperatively.

A cystoscopy can be performed before the initiation of the procedure. It is always useful, especially for beginners, to evaluate the presence of a median lobe and to locate the ureteral orifices. When previous transurethral resection of the prostate has been performed the insertion of double-pigtail catheters is advisable.

4.4 Special Cases for Advanced Surgeons

1. Obesity
2. Prior abdominal surgery
3. Prior inguinal hernia repair with mesh placement
4. Prior transurethral resection of the prostate
5. Very large prostate
6. Presence of large middle lobe
7. Asymmetric prostate
8. Extensive pelvic fibrosis (gunshot injury, orthopedic or trauma surgery)
9. Salvage prostatectomy after brachytherapy, external beam radiation and high-intensity focused ultrasound (HIFU).

4.5 Obesity

Obesity is an increasing health issue and a burden for the public health system. Recent studies reported an age-adjusted prevalence of approximately 20–25% in the German population [4]. Almost 2% of people are is morbidly obese, i.e. have a BMI of at least 40 kg/m2 [4]. Among the best-known obesity-linked diseases are diabetes mellitus, hypertension and cancer, especially breast cancer. In the latter, obesity is a well-known risk factor linked with poorer prognosis. However, the relationship between obesity and prostate cancer is not completely clear. A growing number of studies suggest that the risk of developing prostate cancer as well as the probability of higher-grade disease and disease progression after radical prostatectomy increases with increased BMI. In contrast, an equal number of studies propose a weak association or none at all [5, 6]. Only few reports are available on radical prostatectomy in obese patients [7–10].

In a recent study from our center (unpublished data) we documented that obesity is not a contraindication for EERPE. Indeed, EERPE/nsEERPE can be safely accomplished in obese patients. Increased perioperative complications and intraoperative blood loss in patients with a high BMI can be avoided by performing surgery with adequate consideration and accuracy, at the cost of a slight increase in operation time.

In our view, obese patients (Fig. 4.1) especially benefit from a minimally invasive procedure, since wound healing represents a potential hazard in open surgery. The trocars are inserted more caudally, as described in Chap. 7. In addition, there is a consensus among laparoscopists that the extraperitoneal is more beneficial than the transperitoneal access in these patients.

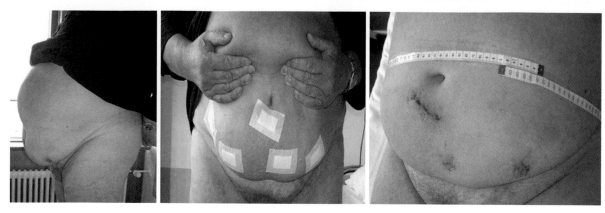

Fig. 4.1. Postoperative appearance of an obese patient

4.6 Prior Abdominal Surgery

Little is known about the effect of previous surgery on the results of laparoscopy. Seifman et al. reported that previous abdominal surgery increased the overall risk of transperitoneal laparoscopic renal and adrenal surgery [11]. In contrast, Parsons et al. described no adverse effect of previous abdominal surgery on the subsequent performance of predominantly laparoscopic renal surgery [12]. While extensive transabdominal surgery or previous pelvic surgery has been regarded as a contraindication for laparoscopic prostatectomy by some authors [13], previous major abdominal surgery or pelvic surgery is not seen as a contraindication per se by others [14]. Nevertheless, in a detailed analysis of perioperative complications by the latter group, the effect of previous intra-abdominal surgery and urological surgery was not clearly stated [15].

In a recent study from our center we analyzed the impact of previous surgery on EERPE. 500 patients who underwent EERPE for clinically localized prostate cancer between December 2001 and April 2004 were stratified into five groups: (I) no previous abdominal, inguinal or prostate surgery; (II) previous upper abdominal surgery; (IIIa) previous lower abdominal or pelvic surgery/open inguinal hernioplasty; (IIIb) laparoscopic/endoscopic inguinal hernioplasty; (IV) previous prostatic surgery and (V) a combination of groups II, III and/or IV. Groups I and II were analyzed together since the previous operative fields in group II were distant from the Retzius space. The operative times, complications and re-interventions were analyzed with the Mann–Whitney, chi-square and Fisher tests. A total of 335 patients (67%) were in groups I–II and 165 patients (33%) in groups III–V. The mean overall operative time was 149±30 min. Four patients (0.8%) required transfusions, with no conversion to open surgery and no mortality. A total of 78 complications (15.6%) and 11 re-interventions (2.2%) occurred. EERPE was subjectively more demanding and challenging in patients with previous minimally invasive hernioplasty with mesh placement. No statistically significant difference was detected between no surgery (groups I–II) and previous surgery (groups III–V) in terms of overall operative time, complications or re-interventions.

Autopsy studies have shown intra-abdominal adhesions after open abdominal surgery in up to 90% of patients [16], while adhesions seem to be less extensive after laparoscopic surgery [17]. In our experience, despite the fact that 35.6% of our patients had undergone previous surgery, we were able to establish standard trocar placement and correct access to the extraperitoneal space of Retzius in all patients, and all procedures could be completed without conversions. We feel that the extraperitoneal route of access contributes significantly to our findings that previous abdominal surgery does not complicate EERPE.

Figure 4.2 shows the postoperative outcome in two patients with prior abdominal surgery. Transperitoneal access would require cumbersome adhesion dissection before the initiation of the actual prostatectomy procedure and significantly increase the risk of complications. Extraperitoneal access avoids these problems. In most cases trocar positioning should be adapted according to the presence of the abdominal scar (see Chap. 7)

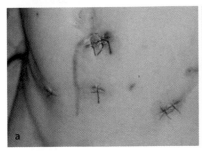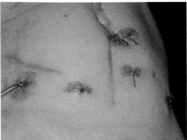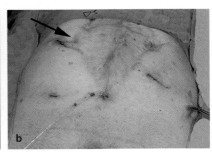

Fig. 4.2. Postoperative appearance of two patients with extensively performed previous pelvic surgery. **a** A patient with two previously performed laparotomies for a perforated appendicitis. **b** A patient with previous abdominal surgery for colon carcinoma. He developed peritonitis and three reinterventions were performed. The insertion of a mesh was deemed necessary to close the fascias and wound after the reinterventions, displacing the umbilicus (*arrow*)

4.7 Prior Inguinal Hernia Repair with Mesh Placement

Inguinal hernia repair is one of the most commonly performed surgical procedures. Laparoscopic inguinal hernia repair preceded the development of laparoscopic radical prostatectomy (LRPE) and is currently available in most specialized centers worldwide. It is inevitable that some candidates for LRPE or EERPE will have a previous history of minimally invasive inguinal hernia repair, in the form of either total extraperitoneal hernioplasty (TEP) or transabdominal extraperitoneal hernioplasty (TAPP). The key element for tension-free herniorrhaphy in TEP or TAPP is the use of prosthetic mesh, which can lead to extensive adhesion between the abdominal wall and the peritoneum. For LRPE or laparoscopic pelvic lymphadenectomy, previous TEP or TAPP with mesh placement has been considered a relative contraindication to laparoscopic surgery or a reason for conversion to open surgery [4, 5]. Our experience has, however, shown that EERPE is feasible in patients with previous TEP or TAPP.

It is inevitable that laparoscopic surgeons will encounter patients who have had hernia repairs performed with an open surgical technique. As the mesh is placed superficially to the transversalis fascia there is no expected difficulty in creating the extraperitoneal space. Indeed, such patients have been operated on in our institution, and surgery could be completed by means of the standard EERPE technique with no difficulty in port placement or the creation of an extraperitoneal space [19].

Some tips and tricks for the management of these patients are described in Chap. 7. The position of the trocars must be adapted according to the adhesions that are present. The patient must be informed that lymphadenectomy is extremely difficult or impossible on the side of the mesh. This is due to the size of the mesh. There are different techniques of mesh placement for hernia repair, but the majority of surgeons tend to use a large mesh overlapping the iliac vessels and the obturator fossa.

4.8 Prior Transurethral Resection of the Prostate

Prior transurethral resection of the prostate (TURP) can make the case more challenging. Clinical experience has proven that there is a wide variation in TURP technique and in the amount of tissue resected. In addition, the bladder neck is resected more aggressively by some surgeons than others. When the bladder neck has been extensively resected, the extent of scar formation can make it extremely challenging to define the border between bladder neck and prostate and to identify the ureteral orifices. Preoperative cystoscopic clarification of the shape of the prostate and the ureteral orifices is suggested. Furthermore, we recommend double-pigtail insertion during the preoperative cystoscopic evaluation. This provides a more secure bladder neck dissection in these patients. The double-pigtail stents can be extracted either after completion of the posterior part of the urethrovesical anastomosis or after the urethral catheter has been extracted (5th postoperative day).

4

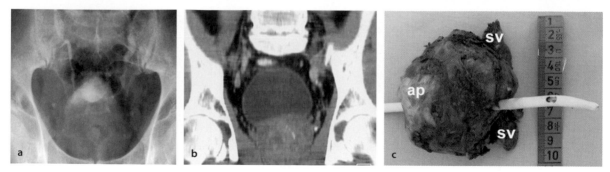

Fig. 4.3. a Intravenous urography and **b** computerized tomography of a patient with a 210-g prostate managed with EERPE. **c** The specimen

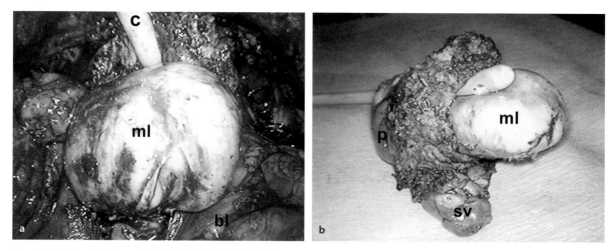

Fig. 4.4. a View of a large middle lobe during EERPE. **b** The specimen

4.9 Atypical Size and Shape of Prostate (Large Prostate – Large Middle Lobe Asymmetric Prostate)

It is known that very small (<30 g) as well as very large prostates represent a challenge for open as well as laparoscopic/endoscopic prostatectomy. Based on our personal experience we would suggest that prostates with a size of 100–150 g should not be selected during the learning curve of a surgeon. Prostates larger than 150 g (or even over 200 g; see Fig. 4.3) should be managed only by experienced surgeons. Especially the posterior apical dissection can be very demanding because of the size of the specimen. This has to be performed in a mixture of a descending and ascending

fashion. There is no special trick that can be suggested for the procedure. One should meticulously follow the steps of standard EERPE.

The size of the middle lobe of the prostate varies from very small to very large (Fig. 4.4). A cystoscopic evaluation before the procedure is suggested to determine the dimensions of the middle lobe. For beginners we would suggest the insertion of double-pigtail catheters to ascertain the integrity of the ureteral orifices during posterior bladder neck dissection. If difficulties are encountered during bladder neck dissection, do not hesitate to open a wider bladder neck and better identify the middle lobe and the anatomy of the bladder neck. When ureteral stenting is not performed, intravenous injection of indigocarmine and

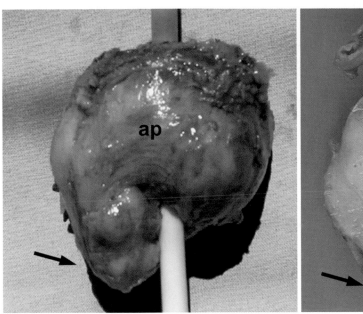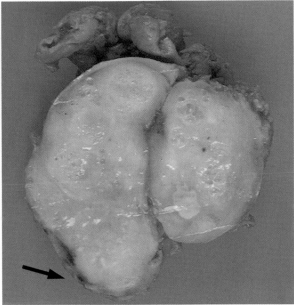

Fig. 4.5. Asymmetric prostate specimen. The tumor has extended towards the apex on the right side (arrow) altering the homogeneous apical prostatic morphology

furosemide is an option to facilitate orifice identification. For an experienced surgeon the presence of a middle lobe should not be a problem. With increasing experience we no longer insert double-pigtail catheters.

An asymmetric prostate can be technically very challenging especially when the anatomical peculiarity is adjacent to the apex. Figure 4.5 shows a rare case where the tumor has extended towards the apex on the right side, altering the homogeneous apical prostatic morphology. The surgeon should be aware of this possibility and identify such special conditions preoperatively with the aid of transrectal ultrasonography.

4.10 Extensive Pelvic Fibrosis

Previous pelvic injury or intervention can cause massive fibrosis, making the procedure demanding. We present two special cases where massive fibrosis was found during surgery. Figure 4.6a shows postprostatectomy cystograms in a patient who was shot with a machine gun in the pelvic area 20 years before prostatectomy. The bullets are clearly seen in the X-rays.

Figure 4.6b shows a postprostatectomy cystogram in a patient who had previous orthopedic surgery after pubic bone fracture due to a motorbike accident. In both patients the prostatectomy was technically demanding due to the massive fibrotic tissue reaction in the pelvic area. The classic resection planes could not be developed, and only sharp dissection was performed during the entire procedure.

4.11 Salvage Prostatectomy After Brachytherapy, External Beam Radiation and HIFU

During the past few decades, various minimally invasive alternative therapies have been developed with the aim of being as efficient as surgical therapy while minimizing side effects and complications. Some of the recently developed therapies are cryosurgical ablation of the prostate, HIFU and radiofrequency interstitial tumor ablation (RITA). These approaches are categorized in the European Association of Urology guidelines as experimental local treatments of prostate cancer [1].

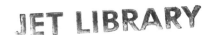

4

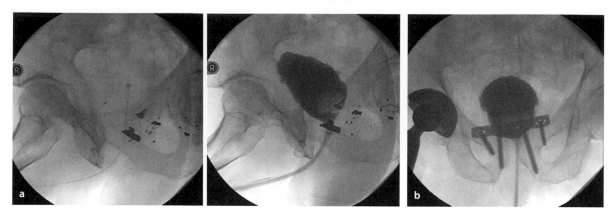

Fig. 4.6. a, b Postprostatectomy cystogram in a patient with previous machine gun injury before prostatectomy. **c** Postpros-tatectomy cystogram in a patient with previous orthopedic surgery after pubic bone fracture and right hip replacement

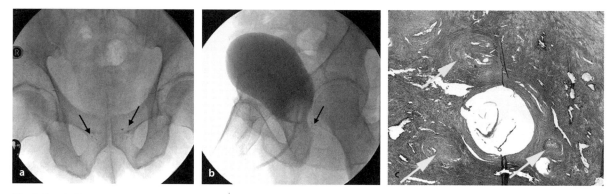

Fig. 4.7. a, b Postoperative cystogram of a patient with previous brachytherapy treatment (1.5 years preoperatively). Note the presence of numerous seeds even postoperatively (*arrows*), documenting their migration into the periprostatic area. **c** The pathology evaluation of the specimen. Carcinoma (*arrows*) was found very close to the former seed site (*white hole*)

Most recurrent or persistent prostate cancers after failed HIFU or radiotherapy are discovered at an early stage due to the wide use of prostatic-specific antigen (PSA) as a marker for monitoring treatment response. For patients in good general condition with a life expectancy greater than 10 years, salvage radical prostatectomy is an option, but it is associated with significant morbidity [20, 21].

We recently investigated the feasibility, efficacy and oncological and short-term functional results of EERPE as a salvage procedure for recurrent prostate cancer after HIFU or radiotherapy (unpublished results). Figure 4.7 shows the postoperative cystogram and pathology evaluation after EERPE in a patient who had undergone brachytherapy 1.5 years previously.

In our series of the first 1,000 EERPEs, nine patients underwent salvage EERPE with curative intent for biopsy-proven locally recurrent prostate cancer. Perioperative parameters (operation time, estimated blood loss, rate of conversion to open surgery, transfusion rate, transurethral catheter time), functional outcome and short-term oncological outcome were reviewed.

The patients' mean age was 63.3 years (range 48–74 years). Mean preoperative PSA was 12.64 ng/ml, and mean prostate weight was 49.2 g. Mean blood loss was 238 ml. There was no need for conversion to open surgery or transfusion. Mean operation time was 148 min, and mean total transurethral catheter time was 6 days. No intraoperative complications were reported. There was no clear difference in difficulty of surgery between post-HIFU and post-radiotherapy EERPE. After a mean follow-up of 17 months, seven patients were completely continent and two needed 1–2 pads a day. Three patients were potent before the surgical treatment but no patient reported potency postoperatively. Only in one patient was a PSA relapse (1.20 ng/ml) recognized 12 months postoperatively.

We thus concluded that salvage EERPE after failed HIFU and radiation therapy is a safe and efficient method to treat locally recurrent prostate cancer. Short-term oncological and functional outcomes are promising but further study should be made on the long-term oncological outcomes.

References

1. Aus G, Abbou CC, Bolla M et al. EAU guidelines on prostate cancer (ISBN 90-70244-27-6) or on the website of the European Association of Urology: http://www.uroweb.org/
2. Simon MA, Kim S, Soloway MS (2006) Prostate-specific antigen recurrence rates are low after radical retropubic prostatectomy and positive margins. J Urol 17:140–144
3. Burkhard FC, Kessler TM, Fleischmann A, Thalmann GN, Schumacher M, Studer UE (2006) Nerve sparing open radical retropubic prostatectomy – does it have an impact on urinary continence? J Urol 176:189–195
4. Deutsche Gesellschaft für Ernährung (2004) Ernährungsbericht 2004. Druckerei Heinrich, Frankfurt am Main
5. Mallah KN, DiBlasio CJ, Rhee AC, Scardino PT, Kattan MW (2005) Body mass index is weakly associated with, and not a helpful predictor of, disease progression in men with clinically localized prostate carcinoma treated with radical prostatectomy. Cancer 103:2030–2034
6. Lee IM, Sesso HD, Paffenbarger RS Jr (2001) A prospective cohort study of the physical activity and body size in relation to prostate cancer risk (United States). Cancer Causes Control 12:187–193
7. Singh A, Fagin R, Shah G, Shekarriz B (2005) Impact of prostate size and body mass index on perioperative mobidity after laparoscopic radical prostatectomy. J Urol 173:552–554
8. Brown JA, Rodin DM, Lee B, Dahl DM (2005) Laparoscopic radical prostatectomy and body mass index: an assessment of 151 sequential cases. J Urol 173:442–445
9. Ahlering TE, Eichel L, Edwards R, Skarecky DW (2005) Impact of obesity on clinical outcomes in robotic prostatectomy. Urology 65:740–744
10. Dahm P, Yang BK, Salmen CR, Moul JW, Gan TJ (2005) Radical perineal prostatectomy for the treatment of localized prostate cancer in morbidly obese patients. J Urol 174:131–134
11. Seifman BD, Dunn RL, Wolf JS Jr (2003) Transperitoneal laparoscopy into the previously operated abdomen: effect on operative time, length of stay and complications. J Urol 169:36–40
12. Parsons JK, Jarrett TJ, Chow GK et al. (2002) The effect of previous abdominal surgery on urological laparoscopy. J Urol 168:2387–2390
13. Rassweiler J, Sentker L, Seemann O et al. (2001) Laparoscopic radical prostatectomy with the Heilbronn technique: an analysis of the first 180 cases. J Urol 166:2101–2108
14. Guillonneau B, Vallancien G (2000) Laparoscopic radical prostatectomy: the Montsouris experience. J Urol 163:418–422
15. Guillonneau B, Rozet F, Cathelineau X et al. (2002) Perioperative complications of laparoscopic radical prostatectomy: the Montsouris 3-year experience. J Urol 167:51–56
16. Weibel MA, Majno G (1973) Peritoneal adhesions and their relation to abdominal surgery. A postmortem study. Am J Surg 126:345–353
17. Pattaras JG, Moore RG, Landman J et al. (2002) Incidence of postoperative adhesion formation after transperitoneal genitourinary laparoscopic surgery. Urology 59:37–41
18. Stolzenburg J-U, Ho K, Do M, Rabenalt R, Dorschner W, Truss MC (2005) Impact of previous surgery on endoscopic extraperitoneal radical prostatectomy (EERPE). Urology 65:325–331
19. Stolzenburg J-U, Anderson C, Rabenalt R, Do M, Ho K, Truss M (2005) Endoscopic extraperitoneal radical prostatectomy (EERPE) in patients with prostate cancer and previous laparoscopic inguinal mesh placement for hernia repair. World J Urol 27:1–5
20. Chen BT, Wood DP (2003) Salvage prostatectomy in patients who have failed radiation therapy or cryotherapy as primary treatment for prostate cancer. Urology 62:69–78
21. Gheiler EL, Tefilli MV, Tiguert R et al. (1998) Predictors for maximal outcome in patients undergoing salvage surgery for radio-recurrent prostate cancer. Urology 51:789–795

Anaesthesia Considerations in Radical Prostatectomy

5

Fritjoff Koenig · Bernd Aedtner · Markus Wehner · Robert Rabenalt · Paraskevi Katsakiori ·
Kriton Filos · Evangelos N. Liatsikos · Jens-Uwe Stolzenburg

Contents

5

5.1 Introduction

The management of anaesthesia in laparoscopic and endoscopic radical prostatectomy can be quite complex. Many surgeons, especially at the beginning of their learning curve, experience difficulties with the anaesthesiologic aspects of the procedure. These problems can be easily managed with proper standardised protocols. Even long operating times in difficult cases can be managed without cardiopulmonary limitations.

Carbon dioxide is currently the most widely applied gas in laparoscopy, but it is absorbed from the peritoneum and retroperitoneum and may cause hypercarbia and acidosis. When the patient is monitored and ventilated under control, hyperventilation may prevent hypercarbia. Currently available insufflators maintain intra-abdominal pressure within pre-programmed values. Only minor haemodynamic changes can occur when the pressure is maintained below 18 mmHg [1–7].

5.2 Contraindications for Anaesthesia

There are only a few contraindications for anaesthesia in LRPE and EERPE. Absolute contraindications are elevated intracranial pressure or non-treatable disorders of coagulation. Advanced stages of heart failure, severe chronic obstructive pulmonary diseases, elevated intrapulmonary shunts and a ventriculoperitoneal shunt are relative contraindications [8–10]. Anaesthesia in these patients may require extended monitoring and postanaesthetic care. Surgery should be delayed for at least 6 weeks in patients with a recent myocardial infarction or a percutaneous coronary intervention with implantation of coronary stents, to avoid re-infarction or a deleterious stent thrombosis.

5.3 Type of Anaesthesia

EERPE is performed under general anaesthesia with intubation of the trachea to avoid aspiration of gastric content. Epidural anaesthesia is not needed because of the minimally invasive character of the procedure and the low level of pain in the postoperative period. Generally, the preferred indications for epidural-based anaesthetic–analgesic techniques in urologic surgery are cystectomy and ileal conduit or neo-blad-

der formation. In these kinds of operation, the sympathetic blockade produces less operative interference with intestinal perfusion and motility (i.e. postoperative bowel paralysis) [10].

5.4 Positioning of the Patient

Gradually acquired experience in the anaesthesiologic aspect of EERPE resulted in modification of the patient position. Initially, the patient was placed in a dorsal supine position with his legs slightly apart while the head was tilted 25° down. As experience increased, we realised that such an extreme Trendelenburg position was not necessary because the bowel did not interfere with the procedure. Thus, 10° head down tilt seems sufficient. No head oedema is observed with less head-down tilt than LPRE.

The patient is completely covered with sterile surgical drapes and supported with a chest belt. Both arms should be well protected by positioning them on the patient's body (see Chap. 7). The surgeon stands to the left of the patient with an assistant opposite, while the camera-holder is positioned behind the head of the patient. The torso and the legs of the patient are draped on the operating table, minimising the risk of movement of the patient during the procedure. Even if any intra-operative change of the patient's position on the operative table occurs, it does not represent a significant problem, due to the diminished head-down tilt. The left arm is always accessible by the anaesthesiologist and the intravenous cannulae are inserted therein. The right arm is draped adherent to the patient's body.

5.5 Monitoring of the Patient

A central line is not necessary and only two peripheral venous lines are placed. An arterial line for invasive monitoring of blood pressure is required only in individuals with advanced cardiopulmonary disease. The basic monitoring includes ECG, non-invasive blood pressure (RR), SaO_2 and inspired/expired O_2 and CO_2 concentration. A relaxometer should be available at the workplace. Insertion of a nasogastric tube (moderate head-down position, extraperitoneal access) is not needed. Because the patient's whole body is covered with sterile tape there is only a minor risk of hypothermia. However, body temperature

Fig. 5.1. Intraoperative changes in end-expiratory partial pressure of CO_2 in EERPE. *Triangles*, initial CO_2 pressure; *squares*, maximum CO_2 pressure

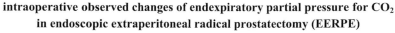

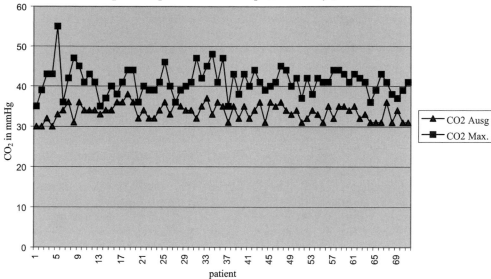

should be assessed at least once at the end of the procedure.

Accurate monitoring of urine output cannot be achieved. Interruptions to the urinary tract and urine flow during the procedure make it unrealistic. Besides, measurement of blood loss is not reliable, because the aspirate is a mixture of blood and urine.

5.6 Pharmaceutical Agents Used During Anaesthesia

General anaesthesia is accomplished by continuous administration of intravenous opiates (i.e. alfentanil 30–50 µg/kg/h) and volatile anaesthetics (i.e. isoflurane) along with endotracheal intubation. Generally, additional muscle relaxation after intubation of the trachea is not necessary, except in the occasional case with increased lung compliance or if the surgeon requires it.

A balanced anaesthesia technique rather than a total intravenous technique is preferred to avoid intraoperative awareness of the patient by disconnection or blocking of the intravenous lines and the reduced access to the patient. Moreover, the balanced technique ensures the monitoring of the expired anaesthetic gases. Intraoperative anaesthesia-related prob-

lems may occur, so fast access to the patient must be guaranteed. A brief interruption of the operation may be necessary. However, good interdisciplinary cooperation should overcome these problems.

Crystalloid solutions for infusion are employed for intraoperative volume substitution. Colloidal solutions are rarely administered and in a volume of less than 500 ml. The average total infusion volume used is reduced to 5 ml/kg/h. No more erythrocyte concentrates are routinely cross-matched, due to the low blood transfusion rate (in our experience of 1,400 EERPEs: intraoperatively 0%, postoperatively 0.9%).

5.7 Ventilation

The mechanical ventilation is pressure-controlled, and is supplemented with an initial positive end-expiratory pressure (PEEP) of 5 mmHg. After insufflation of CO_2 into the extraperitoneal space the lung compliance is impaired and the inspiratory pressure has to be increased. The difference between inspiratory and expiratory pressure levels should usually not exceed 20 mmHg (maximally 25 mmHg). When during the operation this pressure difference is achieved, the PEEP level is titrated by slowly increasing it without changing the pressure difference. The PEEP level that leads to the highest tidal volume is kept constant in order to reduce the pressure difference. In general, we aim for tidal volumes of 6–8 ml/kg, respiration rate of 12–16/min and an inspiratory:expiratory (I:E) ratio of 1:1.5. When using this approach the end-expiratory CO_2 increase can be maintained within justifiable limits. Only in a few patients with a significant end-tidal CO_2 increase (~ 50 mmHg; seen only with long operation times) is the ventilation frequency initially increased to 24–28/min. Nevertheless, in some cases, very high end-expiratory CO_2 values are achieved, which can be more easily tolerated (permissive hypercapnia) (Fig. 5.1).

If problems (i.e. bleeding complications) occur during the operation the pressure is increased by the surgeon up to 20 mmHg. This should be applied only in close coordination with the anaesthetist, since it is always associated with difficulty regarding mechanical ventilation and may last for only a short time (10–15 min).

5.8 Postoperative Pain

In a recent study by Hoznek et al., the mean dose of morphine and the mean duration of its administration was 53.1% and 44.4% lower, respectively, after extraperitoneal than after transperitoneal radical prostatectomy. Although the difference was not statistically significant, the authors considered it clinically relevant. In addition, abdominal tenderness and shoulder pain, commonly observed among LRPE patients, were not reported in their extraperitoneal series [11].

Our initial experience with "minimally invasive treatment" of prostate cancer includes 70 cases performed transperitoneally in 2000 and 2001. Due to the lack of experience at that time we postoperatively transferred all patients to the intensive care unit. Administration of analgesia was started intraoperatively, with a peripherally acting analgesic (metamizole 1–2 g) and continued postoperatively using a patient-controlled analgesia (PCA) pump (with piritramide). Later, the PCA pumps were omitted due to the fact that self-administered bolus doses and the total quantities of the opiates were small.

In December 2001 we completely changed the technique to a completely extraperitoneal access. The patients no longer had to be postoperatively trans-ported to the ICU. They were postoperatively monitored in a postanaesthetic care unit (PACU) or intermediate care unit, although they could have been observed in a regular recovery room. With increasing experience, it became obvious that there is no need for a PCA pump and regular administration of analgesics.

5.9 Role of Carbon Dioxide

Retroperitoneal insufflation of CO_2 is used in several urological procedures despite the potential risk of CO_2 accumulation. The retroperitoneal space offers less of a barrier to CO_2 diffusion than the peritoneum, it is very vascular, it contains adipose tissue and, unlike the peritoneal cavity, it is not a limited cavity. These features result in greater absorption of CO_2 during retroperitoneal than during intraperitoneal laparoscopy.

In certain studies, there was a difference in the extent of CO_2 absorption during retroperitoneoscopy, compared with intraperitoneal laparoscopy. In an experimental pig model, the increase of CO_2 pressure was independent of the intra- or retroperitoneal gas insufflation [7]. On the contrary, in an experimental dog model, the absorption of CO_2 was greater after intra- than after extraperitoneal insufflation [12].

In humans, some authors did not observe greater absorption of CO_2 in retroperitoneoscopic renal surgery than in transperitoneal laparoscopy [13]. However, others found that CO_2 absorption was greater in patients when the retroperitoneal approach instead of the transperitoneal one was used in renal surgery [14]. In addition, Streich et al. reported that retroperitoneal CO_2 insufflation results in more CO_2 absorption than peritoneal insufflation. Persistence of absorption of CO_2 after the end of surgery was observed [3].

Large variations in CO_2 production can be observed during retroperitoneoscopic surgery. Proper management of the ventilator could maintain end-tidal CO_2 within normal values, risking a change in lung volumes and dead space that could affect the alveolo-arterial CO_2 difference.

It is a fact that CO_2 output remained high after retroperitoneoscopy while CO_2 output decreased immediately on cessation of peritoneal insufflation. Persistent accumulation of CO_2 during the early postoperative period should be considered in the postoperative care of patients after retroperitoneoscopy.

Anaesthesia Considerations in Radical Prostatectomy

An additional CO_2 pressure effect on the cerebral circulation is caused in patients in Trendelenburg position for prostate and bladder surgery. A rise in CO_2 blood tension increases cerebral blood flow, whereas intra-abdominal pressure and central haemodynamic effects reduce cerebral blood flow. In addition to an osmotic diuresis towards the end of the procedure, the routine for the prolonged head-down position included restricted fluid loads and maintenance while so positioned. Increases in ventilation rates adjust the rises in end-tidal CO_2.

5.10 Summarised Recommendation

Co-operation between the surgeon and the anaesthesiologist is of paramount importance for safe and effective performance of EERPE. Appropriate anaesthetic equipment and trained personnel must be available. In Table 5.1 we present a brief but meticulous description of the entire anaesthesiological management of the EERPE patient.

Table 5.1. Standardised anaesthesiological management of EERPE

1. Preoperative visit
Preoperative day
- Patient history
- Physical status
- Information of patient about specific content of operation and anaesthesia details (only general anaesthesia is performed; additional regional anaesthesia is not needed due to low postoperative pain)
- Twelve-lead electrocardiogram
- Laboratory investigations (basic blood test, electrolytes, coagulation status, glucose)
- Chest X-ray, spirometry, echocardiography only in cases with severe cardiac or pulmonary comorbidities
- In night before operation, administration of long-acting benzodiazepines (e.g. 5 mg nitrazepam or 1 mg flunitrazepam)
- Prophylaxis of thromboembolic events with fractionated heparin (replacement of pre-existing long-acting medication with short-acting anticoagulatory agents; interruption of acetylsalicylic acid intake for 3–5 days)

Operative day
- Continuation of comedications
- Premedication with midazolam (5–10 mg p.o. 1 h before anaesthesia initiation)

2. In the operating room
Patient positioning
- Supine position
- Right arm: noninvasive blood pressure measurement. Arm is attached to body and fixed under a sheath (no arm holder; fixation of this arm should be performed when patient is conscious to prevent inadvertent nerve injuries)
- Left arm: SaO_2 measurement. One intravenous cannula preoperatively, and one after induction of anesthesia. Elongation of infusion line with injection port to upper end of table. Arm is positioned on arm holder fixed to operating table (use of silicone protective gel)
- ECG (standard leads; if needed, additional leads II and V5 for detection of ischemic events)
- Extended monitoring (invasive arterial blood pressure measurement only in patients with high cardiac risk; temperature measurement and rewarming blankets only if needed)
- Belt with a silicone protective sheath under it, on upper part of thorax (prevent movement of patient during operation in the case of extreme Trendelenburg positioning); never use mechanical restraints on shoulder area because of danger to plexus brachialis

Anaesthesia
Induction
- Opioid injection (i.e. 20–30 µg/kg alfentanil)
- Induction with 1.5–2 mg/kg propofol (in the case of pre-existing cardiac comorbidities or hypotensive patients, 0.2–0.3 mg/kg etomidate is preferable)
- Relaxation (i.e. 0.6 mg/kg rocuronium)
- Intubation with RAE tube; connection with extension (patient's head is not accessible during operation; safe positioning protecting airway system on patient's head; avoidance of pressure damage to patient's face; eye protection by ointment)

Continuation as balanced anaesthesia
- Isoflurane or desflurane with O_2/air mixture (FiO_2 0.4)

Table 5.1. (Continued)

- Optimised ventilation monitoring is performed and the supply of the narcotic agent is provided by the volatile anaesthetic. When intravenous method is applied, supply of anaesthetic can be interrupted because of poor access to long infusion lines.
- Continuation of opiates (i.e. 30–60 µg/kg/h alfentanil) until beginning or end of anastomosis (depending on speed of suturing by surgeon)
- Intermittent relaxation if needed (TOF monitoring of muscle relaxation)
- Ventilation
  - Pressure controlled
  - PEEP = 5 mbar
  - Ventilator frequency 10–14 per minute
  - Time inspiration/expiration (t_i:t_E) = 1:1.5
  - Pressure difference between P_{exp} and P = 20 mbar
- In the case of CO_2 increase
  - Elevation of minute volume with increase of ventilatory frequency
  - If ineffective, increase of PEEP with same pressure difference
  - The level of PEEP is titrated to have a tidal volume of 6–8 ml/kg body weight
  - The pressure difference between expiratory and inspiratory is increased to maximal 25 mbar
  - Reduction of CO_2 insufflation pressure (decrease in intra-abdominal pressure)
  - If CO_2 is continuously increasing, high CO_2 values are tolerated (risk/benefit balance)

Recovering from anaesthesia
- Extubation in operating room
- Transport with O_2 insufflation via face mask or nasal line and monitoring to intermediate care unit (at least SaO_2)

3. **Postoperatively**
- Pain therapy with non-opioid analgesics, e.g. paracetamol (acetaminophen) or metamizol, and rarely opioids, e.g. piritramide on demand

References

1. Drummond GB, Duncan MK (2002) Abdominal pressure during laparoscopy: effects of fentanyl. Br J Anaesth 88:384–388
2. Seed RF, Shakespeare TF, Muldoon MJ (1970) Carbon dioxide homeostasis during anaesthesia for laparoscopy. Anaesthesia 25:223–231
3. Streich B, Decailliot B, Perney C, Duvaldestin P (2003) Increased carbon dioxide absorption during retroperitoneal laparoscopy. Br J Anaesth 91:793–796
4. Hodgson C, McClelland RMA, Newton JR (1970) Some effects of the peritoneal insufflation of carbon dioxide at laparoscopy. Anaesthesia 25:382–390
5. Baird JE, Granger R, Klein R, Warriner CB, Phang PT (1999) The effects of peritoneal carbon dioxide insufflation on hemodynamics and arterial carbon dioxide. Am J Surg 177:164–166
6. Hirvonen EA, Poikolainen EO, Paakkonen ME, Nuutinen LS (2000) The adverse hemodynamic effects of anesthesia, head-up tilt, and carbon dioxide pneumoperitoneum during laparoscopic cholecystectomy. Surg Endosc 14:272–277
7. Coskun F, Salman MA (2001) Anesthesia for operative endoscopy. Curr Opin Obstet Gynecol 13:371–376
8. Stolzenburg J-U, Rabenalt R, Do M, Ho K, Dorschner W, Waldkirch E, Jonas U, Schütz A, Horn L, Truss MC (2005) Endoscopic extraperitoneal radical prostatectomy (EE-RPE) – oncological and functional results after 700 procedures. J Urol 174:1271–1275
9. Stolzenburg J-U, Truss MC (2003) Technique of laparoscopic (endoscopic) radical prostatectomy. BJU Int 91:749–757
10. Stolzenburg JU, Aedtner B, Olthoff D, Koenig F, Rabenalt R, Filos K, McNeill A, Liatsikos EN (2006) Anaesthesia considerations for endoscopic extraperitoneal and laparoscopic transperitoneal radical prostatectomy. BJU Int 98:508–513
11. Hoznek A, Antiphon P, Borkowski T, Gettman MT, Katz R, Salomon L, Zaki S, de la Taille A, Abbou CC (2003) Assessment of surgical technique and perioperative morbidity associated with extraperitoneal versus transperitoneal laparoscopic radical prostatectomy. Urology 61:617–622
12. Wolf JS, Carrier S, Stoller ML (1995) Intraperitoneal versus extraperitoneal insufflation of carbon dioxide as for laparoscopy. J Endourol 9:63–66
13. Ng CS, Gill IS, Sung GT, Whalley DG, Graham R, Schweizer D (1999) Retroperitoneoscopic surgery is not associated with increased carbon dioxide absorption. J Urol 162:1268–1272
14. Wolf JS Jr, Monk TG, McDougall EM, McClennan BL, Clayman RV (1995) The extraperitoneal approach and subcutaneous emphysema are associated with greater absorption of carbon dioxide during laparoscopic renal surgery. J Urol 154:959–963

Pelvic Lymphadenectomy in the Management of Prostate Cancer

6

Sivaprakasam Sivalingam · H. Schwaibold

Contents

6

6.1 Introduction

In the era before prostate-specific antigen (PSA), when patients presented in advanced stages of prostate cancer, pelvic lymphadenectomy was the only available tool to provide staging information prior to commencement of surgical treatment for the prostate cancer. Contemporary imaging modalities such as bilateral pedal lymphangiography lacked sufficient sensitivity to replace surgical lymph-node staging.

With the advent of PSA testing, the emphasis in prostate cancer management shifted gradually from treatment of disease to screening for disease. The increasing recourse to PSA testing and transrectal ultrasound-guided prostate biopsy meant that prostate cancers were diagnosed at earlier stages of their evolution. Medical treatment of prostate cancer with hormones was also beginning to gain momentum. These factors led many clinicians to question the practice of routine pelvic lymphadenectomy for prostate cancer staging. Alternative strategies were devised for selecting patients who required lymph-node staging prior to initiation of treatment. Prognostic tools and nomograms were developed, integrating the patient's individual clinical and histological findings. These tools were then used to select patients with a high risk of lymph-node metastasis for surgical exploration.

The follow-up of patients who developed biochemical recurrence after radical prostatectomy in individual centres suggests that despite low prediction of metastasis by nomograms, these patients may have harboured micrometastasis in their lymph nodes at the time of their initial presentation. This reinvigorated some experts to re-explore the role of „limited" and „extended" pelvic lymphadenectomy in the past few years. Newer developments in surgery such as laparoscopic surgery and robotic surgery have also fuelled this interest in pelvic lymphadenectomy as they offer a minimally invasive procedure which is more acceptable to the patient and promise reduced morbidity compared to the open procedure.

Despite major developments in prostate cancer treatment over the past two decades, the role of pelvic lymphadenectomy in prostate cancer treatment has yet to be clearly defined. Unlike other pelvic malignancies such as colorectal cancer [1] and gynaecological cancer [2], where guidelines exist, prostate cancer lacks any clear consensus on surgical management of pelvic lymph-node disease.

The practice of performing pelvic lymphadenectomy today varies significantly among urological surgeons, with some performing the procedure only in high-risk patients, based on preoperative parameters, while others offer the procedure to all patients undergoing localised treatment of their prostate cancer. The key questions are as follows:

- Does pelvic lymphadenectomy per se alter the prognosis of the disease?
- Which patients should undergo pelvic lymphadenectomy?
- What are the relevant anatomical boundaries for optimal pelvic lymph-node dissection?
- How should the lymph-node tissue be evaluated in the histopathology laboratory?
- Which surgical technique should be used?

In the following sections we discuss these questions, the current practice, its related issues and the scientific evidence behind the rationale for performing pelvic lymphadenectomy in patients with prostate cancer.

6.2 Can Pelvic Lymphadenectomy Alter Prognosis?

The question of whether pelvic lymphadenectomy is a staging tool, or in addition has a therapeutic impact in the era of prostate cancer stage migration and lymph-node micrometastasis, is still unanswered.

Bhatta-Dar et al. retrospectively examined the role of pelvic lymph-node dissection (PLND) in 336 men who underwent radical prostatectomy [3]. In this series, the patients had a PSA level of <10 ng/ml, a Gleason score of <7 and were of clinical stage T1 or T2. They were divided into 140 men who had PLND and 196 men who did not undergo PLND during radical prostatectomy based on the discretion of the operating surgeon. The two groups were evenly matched in terms of age, family history of prostate cancer, race, clinical staging and PSA. The boundaries of the PLND included the external iliac vein, pelvic sidewall, obturator nerve, bifurcation of the common iliac artery and inguinal ligament. The PLND group had a 0.7% metastasis rate in the lymph nodes.

The results showed no statistically significant difference in biochemical relapse rates after a mean follow-up of 60 months. On the multivariate analysis, PLND did not appear to be an independent predictor of the outcome. The estimated 6-year biochemical relapse-free survival rate also showed no statistical significance. This was a retrospective non-randomised study and, in terms of prostate cancer natural history, had a relatively short follow-up interval.

Salomon et al., in a prospective, non-randomised study, compared 43 men with preoperative PSA of <10 ng/ml and a Gleason score of <7 who did not undergo PLND prior to perineal prostatectomy with 25 men with similar PSA and Gleason score who underwent PLND during retropubic prostatectomy [4]. The actuarial 5-year recurrence rates for both groups were not statistically significantly different. Although this was a prospective study, the patient numbers were small and the follow-up interval short. The authors of this study did not describe the surgical dissection template used in the lymphadenectomy procedure, which is crucial, as will be described later.

Both the above studies incorporated only patients with low risk of lymph-node metastasis, based on their preoperative parameters. Such a narrow selection of subjects makes it difficult to draw any conclusion on the efficacy of PLND as a therapeutic modality, as most patients in these studies would have had low risk of lymph-node metastasis anyway.

Bader et al. retrospectively examined the impact of lymph-node metastasis on disease progression and survival [5]. They performed a meticulous lymphadenectomy incorporating the internal, external and obturator lymph-node packets during radical prostatectomy in 367 patients with organ-confined prostate cancer. The preoperative patient selection criteria in terms of PSA level and Gleason grade were broader in this study than in the two studies described above. Ninety-two patients (25%) had histologically proven lymph-node metastasis. Cox regression analysis showed that the probability for PSA relapse, symptomatic progression and tumour-related death increased with each additional lymph node involved. Forty per cent of patients with only one positive lymph node remained without signs of clinical or chemical progression after a follow-up of 45 months.

Frazier et al., in a retrospective analysis of 156 cases from the pre-PSA screening era, showed a similar survival advantage in patients with low-volume pelvic lymph-node involvement [6]. This suggests that not all lymph-node-positive cases automatically have a poor prognosis.

In low-volume lymph-node metastasis, pelvic lymphadenectomy may have a therapeutic impact and confer a survival advantage. In order to demonstrate this point, a prospective multicentre randomised trial recruiting patients with low, medium and high risk of lymph-node metastasis is required. They should all be subjected to a standardised protocol (identical surgical dissection template and technique of histological analysis) during the lymphadenectomy procedure. They should also all receive identical treatments for their prostate cancer and be followed up for at least 10 years. At present, however, there are no such published data to demonstrate the therapeutic impact of pelvic lymphadenectomy.

6.3 Patient Selection for Pelvic Lymphadenectomy

The published literature has recorded an apparent "fall" in lymph-node metastasis rates from 20–40% in the 1970s and 1980s to the present rate of about 6% [7, 8]. This downward pathological stage migration of prostate cancer is thought by many to be secondary to early detection by virtue of PSA screening programs.

Prostate cancer nomograms were developed with the aim of predicting the prognosis in patients with prostate cancer. Partin's Table and the Memorial Sloan Kettering Cancer Center Prostate Nomogram are examples of such tools that have been used to identify preoperatively patients who are at increased risk of lymph-node metastasis [9, 10].

Nomograms are useful in the clinical setting when discussing treatment options with patients as they provide means of quantifying the individual patient's risk in terms of morbidity and mortality. However, their usefulness as an aid for the clinician's decision making has yet to be fully explored. Ross et al. catalogued 42 different types of prostate cancer nomograms in their review in 2001 [11]. They concluded that more comparative studies on the predictive accuracy of the various published nomograms were needed. The authors also felt that more studies comparing the predictive accuracy of nomograms with that of an expert clinician's judgement were necessary. Such comparisons will help determine the true usefulness of prostate cancer nomograms in routine clinical practice.

These nomograms have several drawbacks:
- They rely on results of historical lymphadenectomy series without proper definition of the anatomical boundaries of the lymph-node dissection.

In most cases they rely on a form of limited dissection [8–10].

- Digital rectal examination is subjective and not easily reproducible due to inter-observer variability.
- Discrepancy in Gleason grade exists between Tru-Cut prostate biopsies and the final prostatectomy specimen. Burkhard et al. showed a 24% rate of undergrading and 12% overgrading between Tru-Cut prostate biopsy samples and the final histopathological examination of the radical prostatectomy specimen [12].
- Recent changes in histopathological reporting with a trend towards higher grade assignment means that the Gleason grade data used to establish these prediction nomograms are not comparable to the modern patient [13].

6.4 Anatomical Boundaries in Pelvic Lymphadenectomy

Anatomical dissections and lymphographic studies have demonstrated that prostate lymphatics drain via three pathways [14, 15]:

- Ascending ducts – draining into the external iliac lymph nodes
- Lateral ducts – draining into the hypogastric lymph nodes
- Posterior ducts – draining into the sacral lymph nodes

Schuessler et al. [16] described the various forms of pelvic lymphadenectomies performed on prostate cancer patients (Table 6.1).

The distribution of the pelvic lymph nodes is illustrated in Fig. 6.1.

Bader et al. demonstrated that the anatomical boundaries in lymphadenectomy influence the accuracy of detection of lymph-node metastasis [17]. In their retrospective study, they were able to demonstrate that the sampling of the internal iliac lymph nodes was important. Eighty-eight of the 365 patients in their series had positive lymph nodes. Of these 88 patients, 17 (19%) had positive nodes confined exclusively to the internal iliac area. In an earlier study, McDowell et al. showed a high incidence (29%) of lymph-node metastases also confined exclusively to the internal iliac nodes [18].

Burkhard et al. demonstrated that when a meticulous lymphadenectomy (internal, external iliac and obturator lymph-node packets) was carried out in patients with localised prostate cancer, even "low risk" patients with a PSA level of 10 ng/ml and preoperative cytological grade <3 had a 10% lymph-node metastasis rate [12].

On the other hand, Clark et al.'s prospective randomised evaluation of 123 patients undergoing radical prostatectomy concluded that an extended dissection (common iliac, internal iliac, external iliac, obturator fossa and presacral nodes) does not improve the accuracy of lymph-node staging compared to a limited dissection (external iliac and obturator fossa nodes) [19]. This publication, however, exhibited several shortcomings: its patient population was at low risk of lymph-node metastasis based on preoperative parameters and the patient numbers were too small for an equivalence study. The histopathological evaluation protocol was also not fully described. The randomisation procedure assigned the extended dissec-

Table 6.1. Description of lymphadenectomies by Schuessler in 1993

Terminology	Anatomical boundaries of lymphadenectomy
Standard lymphadenectomy	Common iliac artery, external iliac artery, genitofemoral nerve, hypogastric vessels and obturator fossa nodes
Extended lymphadenectomy	As *standard* plus presacral and lateral sacral nodes
Modified or *limited* lymphadenectomy	Numerous variations:
	As *standard* with omission of common iliac artery, +/– hypogastric vessels and external iliac artery or vein as lateral margin instead of genitofemoral nerve
Obturator fossa lymphadenectomy	Obturator fossa nodes only

Fig. 6.1. Pelvic lymph nodes dissected during pelvic lymphadenectomy

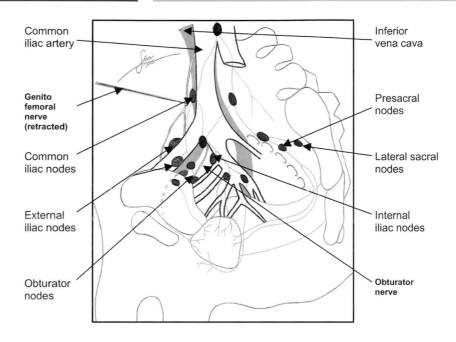

Table 6.2. Lymph-node metastasis pick-up rates from published series

| Series | Extent of lymphadenectomy | | | | |
	Limited	Standard	Modified	Extended	Unclassified
Heidenreich [23] (n=203)		12%		26%	
Parkin [26] (n=50)					24%
Shackley [27] (n=27)					7%
Clark [19] (n=123)	2%			3%	
Allaf [24] (n=4000)	1%			3%	
Stone [25] (n=189)			7%	23%	
Bader [17] (n=365)					24%
Schuessler [16] (n=86)		23%			
Lezin [28] (n=44)					27%
Herrell [21] (n=68)			NA		
Golimbu [22] (n=30)				50%	
McDowell [18] (n=217)					59%

NA, not available

tion only unilaterally, while on the contralateral side a limited dissection was carried out. This meant that the investigators could have potentially missed lymph-node metastasis pick-up from the extended dissection in cases where the prostate cancer focus was only unilateral. These factors can affect the interpretation of the efficacy of the surgical techniques that were compared.

The total number of lymph nodes removed during a lymphadenectomy procedure is of importance in order to maintain the accuracy of the staging procedure. Weingärtner et al. showed through their work on cadaveric pelvic dissections that approximately 20 lymph nodes must be present in the histopathological specimen to ensure an adequate and representative pelvic lymphadenectomy [20].

Examination of current papers on the subject of pelvic lymphadenectomy quickly demonstrates the lack of standardisation in nomenclature and surgical practice. Terminologies such as standard, limited or modified, extended and obturator fossa lymphadenectomy are loosely used to describe the surgical procedure. The anatomical boundaries denoted by these terminologies are inconsistent, as shown by a review of existing publications [16–19, 21–28].

The lymph-node metastasis rates obtained in different lymphadenectomy series are also variable, partly due to the variation in the surgical practice (Table 6.2).

The general lack of consistency creates an unclear picture of the outcomes from the procedure. Therefore, there is a need to reach an international consensus on the standardisation of the anatomical boundaries and establish an agreed nomenclature to describe the surgical boundaries. Surgical lymphadenectomy performed in breast cancer [29] and gastric cancer [30] patients has been stratified into clearly defined levels of surgical dissection. Similar stratification would be invaluable for pelvic lymphadenectomy in prostate cancer and would ensure uniformity of surgical practice. It would also aid in the interpretation and comparison of future studies on pelvic lymphadenectomy in prostate cancer.

6.5 Histopathological Analysis of Pelvic Lymphadenectomy Tissue

The role of frozen section diagnosis in the assessment of pelvic lymph nodes at the time of radical prostatectomy has shown varying use over the last 20 years. In 1986, Epstein et al. reviewed 310 patients, who had had frozen sections and found that the frozen sections detected 67% of positive lymph nodes, which were grossly uninvolved and all the patients with grossly involved lymph nodes [31]. These authors concluded that this was a useful technique in grossly uninvolved nodes. Since that time PSA testing and nomograms predicting positive lymph nodes have been developed. Young et al. in 1999 examined the cost and accuracy of frozen sections before radical prostatectomy and found a false-negative rate of 33% (similar to Epstein et al.) [32]. These authors estimated the cost of metastatic cancer detection to be £7,516 (ca. €11,000). In view of this and the false-negative rate, they concluded that frozen section was not routinely warranted.

Beissner et al. in 2002 found an even higher false-negative rate of 70%, but by stratifying patients into low, intermediate and high risk based on nomograms they improved the sensitivity [33]. They concluded that low-risk patients (stage T2 or less, PSA level of 10 ng/ml or less and Gleason score of 6 or less) gain no benefit from frozen section, whilst the intermediate group (stage T2 or less and Gleason score 7 and/or PSA level of 10.1–20 ng/ml) gain minimal benefit. The high-risk patients who have elected for surgery do gain benefit as they have high risk of positive lymph nodes and detecting such nodes could save them the morbidity of radical prostatectomy.

A variety of histopathological techniques have been used to examine lymph nodes in the laboratory. Pelvic lymph nodes are usually not visible but are palpable and are extensively replaced by adipose tissue, leaving just a small rim of lymphoid tissue at the edge. Some authors feel that this makes these nodes impossible to count accurately [34], whilst others use fat-dissolving techniques (e.g. acetone or xylene) to count them [5, 20]. Fat clearance has been shown to increase lymph-node harvest in colorectal carcinoma [35], but the lymph nodes in the colonic mesentery are well defined and lack the degree of fat infiltration seen in pelvic nodes. This discrepancy makes it impossible to assess surgical technique solely on the basis of the number of lymph nodes harvested by the pathologist.

Studies in colorectal cancers have shown that the more lymph nodes recovered the more accurate the staging [36]. Similar work looking at the pelvic lymph nodes from prostate cancer patients came to the same conclusion [37]. This study showed that the number of lymph nodes recovered varied from 5 to 40, and in those with 13 or more nodes the metastatic lymph-node involvement was twice as high as in those with lower lymph-node counts. Colectomy specimens differ considerably from pelvic lymphadenectomies, as in the latter all the tissues submitted by the surgeon can be blocked and examined, which is not feasible in colectomies. As a result the number of lymph nodes may not be known but the status of all of them is.

When the lymph nodes have been processed and examined, further histopathological techniques can affect the positive rate in the lymph nodes. The positive rate has been shown to increase in colorectal carcinomas with examination of the lymph nodes at several levels [38], and this has also been shown in prostate cancer [39]. Wawroschek et al. showed that by examining lymph nodes at several levels combined with immunohistochemistry the node positive rate in low-risk patients increased from 5% to 11% but there was a smaller increase in the intermediate-risk patients, from 34% to 37%. The cautionary note about using immunohistochemistry to detect micrometastasis is that we are uncertain of the prognostic significance.

It is essential that the histopathological techniques used to detect metastasis are considered when data from various pelvic lymphadenectomy studies are compared.

6.6 Surgical Techniques in Pelvic Lymphadenectomy

Both open and laparoscopic pelvic lymphadenectomy have been described in the literature. Some centres perform laparoscopic pelvic lymphadenectomy before a planned perineal prostatectomy, radical radiotherapy, brachytherapy or cryotherapy.

Lymph-node harvest during laparoscopic lymphadenectomy is comparable to its open counterpart in centres where the learning curve has been overcome [21, 40]. Parkin et al.'s series demonstrated that the laparoscopic procedure has low complication rates [26]. Solberg et al.'s 132 cases (94 open cases and 38 laparoscopic cases) had a significantly lower lymphocele complication rate in the laparoscopic group [41]. Improved magnification and a meticulous need for haemostasis during laparoscopy may be a contributing factor to this observation.

Two routes of laparoscopy are described in the literature: the transperitoneal and the preperitoneal approach. The preperitoneal approach results in less interference from small bowel loops and it mimics the standard open approach. The transperitoneal approach, however, gives better access to the internal iliac and presacral lymph nodes for those who attempt a more extended resection and has a lower lymphocele rate. The latter is due to the communication between the preperitoneal and the intraperitoneal space.

Overhead costs are higher in laparoscopic lymphadenectomy than in its open counterpart [21, 28]. In high-caseload laparoscopic units, however, the costs can be reduced by substituting disposable kits with reusable ones and tailoring laparoscopic kits specifically to the surgeon's requirements so that instruments are not unnecessarily desterilised.

6.7 Sentinel Lymph-Node Mapping in Prostate Cancer

Research has been conducted to determine whether pelvic lymphadenectomy in prostate cancer can be targeted to metastatic lymph nodes, thereby sparing patients the morbidity arising from extensive PLND. This meant that researchers revisited the concept of the 'sentinel lymph node' in the context of prostate cancer.

Wawroschek was among the first to demonstrate the feasibility of sentinel lymph-node (SLN) mapping in prostate cancer patients [42]. Technetium-99m-labelled nanocolloid radio-isotope was injected into each lobe of the prostate under transrectal ultrasound guidance in 348 patients. The 'hot nodes' were then identified with preoperative lymphoscintigraphy and intraoperative gamma probe detection. After the surgical removal of the SLNs (hot nodes), the patients underwent either modified or extended lymphadenectomy based on preoperative risk stratification. The SLN technique demonstrated a metastasis rate of 24%. Most of the histopathologically proven metastatic SLNs were found in the external and internal iliac node packets. The authors concluded that with a pelvic lymphadenectomy confined to the obturator fossa, they would have missed approximately 60% of the metastatic cases in their series.

A recent pilot study on SLN in prostate cancer by Brenot-Rossi et al. showed a 15% metastasis rate [43]. All cases of metastasis involved the SLNs. 50% of the SLNs in this series were distributed along the internal iliac lymph-node packets. The study comprised only 27 men, and the additional surgical lymphadenectomy performed after the removal of the SLN included lymph nodes from the obturator and external iliac region only.

The authors of the first study made no comments on the anatomical boundaries of the comparative pelvic lymphadenectomy, while the authors of the second study did not include the non-SLN internal iliac lymph nodes. This is an important point, as the extent of the dissection directly impacts on the lymph-node metastasis rates.

The SLN mapping technique in prostate cancer has limitations. Unlike breast cancer and melanoma of the skin, it is not possible to "visualise" the tumour within the prostate to deliver a peritumoral injection of the radio-isotope contrast. Therefore, the SLNs identified may not be histopathologically infiltrated with tumour. In practise, this could give rise to false-negative results if the pelvic lymphadenectomy were purely limited to such SLNs. It may not always be possible to get the collimator close enough to SLNs in difficult-to-reach anatomical locations such as the presacral and pararectal regions. It is not known how many of these nodes may have been missed in these studies. In addition, the 'background noise' generated by the prostate might impede the detection of 'hot nodes' in the periprostatic area.

6.8 Imaging Pelvic Lymph Nodes in Prostate Cancer

Radiologists have long sought to find means of determining lymph-node metastasis without subjecting patients to the surgeon's scalpel. Bilateral pedal lymphangiography initially showed promise, but it later became evident that this modality lacked sensitivity [44]. Percutaneous lymph-node biopsy of suspicious radio-opaque lymph nodes on lymphangiography was used as a means of enhancing the sensitivity [45]. This modality eventually gave way to CT in the late 1970s.

At present, the assessment of lymph-node metastasis with imaging modalities such as CT and MRI of the pelvis still lacks sufficient sensitivity to replace the 'gold standard' of surgical lymphadenectomy. Wolf et al. reviewed 25 studies on CT and MRI pelvic imaging which used histopathological confirmation of lymph-node metastasis. They revealed that CT and MRI had a combined sensitivity of only 36% and specificity of 97% in detecting lymph-node metastasis in prostate cancer [46].

Borley et al.'s contemporary series compared the sensitivity and specificity of both CT and MRI with surgical lymphadenectomy in 55 high-risk prostate cancer patients. They found a sensitivity of 27.3% for MRI and 0% for CT [47].

ProstaScint is a technique which utilises capromab pendetide, a monoclonal antibody that specifically targets the prostate-specific membrane antigen. This form of functional imaging is fused with images taken from CT or MRI to provide a detail map of cancer infiltration within the lymph nodes. However, a clinical trial by Ponsky et al. showed a low sensitivity of 17% and specificity of 90% for this modality [48]. The false-positive rate was unacceptably high at 89%. This clinical trial had some limitations: it included only 22 subjects, and the histopathological analysis was surgically limited to obturator fossa and common iliac nodes only.

The utilisation of PET scans in prostate cancer lymph-node staging has been explored with a multitude of tracers. Of these, only [^{11}C]choline or acetate tracer appears to have emerged as suitable for the assessment of lymph nodes [49]. De Jong et al. examined 67 patients with histopathologically proven lymph-node metastasis using [^{11}C]choline PET and demonstrated sensitivity of 80% and specificity of 96% [50]. Although these results are promising, more trials with larger numbers of patients will be needed to confirm and validate these findings.

Intravenous lymphotropic superparamagnetic nanoparticles have been explored in prostate cancer lymph-node staging during MRI scanning. This technique revealed far better sensitivity (90.5% vs 35.4%) and specificity (97.8% vs 90.5%) than the conventional MRI technique in the 80 cases studied [51]. The sensitivity of this technique was, however, low (41.1%) for lymph nodes with diameter <5 mm on the short axis. This is particularly important because patients who have microscopic metastatic disease in the lymphatic sinusoids may be the ones who would benefit the most from a pelvic lymphadenectomy.

In this study, the baseline lymphadenectomy performed for the comparison was rather limited by including only the obturator fossa lymph-node package, except in nine cases where a more extensive exploration was carried out. The sensitivity and specificity of this novel MRI technique may therefore have been overestimated. The findings of this single-centre study also require confirmation before our daily clinical practice is altered as a result.

6.9 Conclusion

The practice of pelvic lymphadenectomy in prostate cancer needs standardisation of both the nomenclature and methodology of the surgical procedure. Patient selection and the technique of histopathological analysis also need to be harmonised. We need standardised protocols to improve our understanding of lymph-node metastasis in prostate cancer. Only this approach will enable us to obtain a better picture of the impact of pelvic lymphadenectomy both in staging and potentially in treatment.

The key question of whether pelvic lymphadenectomy has a therapeutic role in prostate cancer management has not been answered comprehensively. There is some evidence pointing in the same direction as in other cancers, i.e. the smaller the volume of lymph-node metastasis, the better the prognosis. A large retrospective multicentre examination of the long-term biochemical recurrence rates and survival of patients with documented nodal disease after pelvic lymphadenectomy and radical prostatectomy (without adjuvant therapy) is now overdue. Only a detailed analysis of those data can elucidate the role of pelvic lymphadenectomy as a therapeutic modality in prostate cancer.

However, in order to be able to prove or dismiss the concept of therapeutic pelvic lymphadenectomy, a prospective randomised trial would still be necessary. It is unlikely that any future such trial can give us the answer, due to the fact that many patients today undergo localised treatment of their prostate cancer with curative intent although many of them might not succumb to the cancer if it were left untreated. New developments in prostate cancer prognosticators could help us to define the patient population who "truly" need radical treatment and those who might benefit from inclusion of pelvic lymphadenectomy in their treatment protocol.

For the moment, however, each individual clinician will have to decide if and when to perform pelvic lymphadenectomy for patients with prostate cancer.

References

1. Nelson Heidi, Petrelli N, Carlin A, et al (2001) Guidelines 2000 for colon and rectal cancer surgery. J Natl Cancer Inst 93:583–596
2. Benedet JL, Bender H, Jones H 3rd, Ngan HY, Pecorelli S (2000) Staging classification and clinical practice guidelines in the management of gynaecological cancers. FIGO Committee on Gynecologic Oncology. Int J Gynaecol Obstet 70:209–262
3. Bhatta-Dar N, Reuther AM, Zippe C, Klein EA (2004) No difference in six-year biochemical failure rates with or without pelvic lymph-node dissection during radical prostatectomy in low risk patients with localised prostate cancer. Urology 63:528–531
4. Salomon L, Hoznek A, Lefrère-Belda MA, Bellot J, Chopin DK, Abbou CC (2000) Nondissection of pelvic lymph-node does not influence the results of perineal radical prostatectomy in selected patients. Eur Urol 37:297–300
5. Bader P, Burkard FC, Markwalder R, Studer UE (2003) Disease progression and survival of patients with positive after radical prostatectomy. Is there a chance for cure? J Urol 169:849–854
6. Frazier HA 2nd, Robertson JE, Paulson DF (1994) Does radical prostatectomy in the presence of positive pelvic lymph-node enhance survical? World J Urol 12:308–312
7. Fowler JE, Whitmore WF Jr (1981) The incidence and extent of pelvic lymph-node metastases in apparently localised prostate cancer. Cancer 47:2941–2945
8. Partin AW, Kattan MW, Subong EN, et al (1997) Combination of prostate-specific antigen, clinical stage, and Gleason score to predict pathological stage of localised prostate cancer. A multi-institutional update. JAMA 147:1445–1451
9. Partin AW, Mongold LA, Lamm DM, Walsh PC Epstein JI, Pearson JD (2001) Contemporary update of prostate cancer staging nomograms (Partin Tables) for the new millennium. Urology 58:843–848
10. Cagiannos I, Karakiewicz P, Eastham JA, et al (2003) A preoperative nomogram identifying decreased risk of positive pelvic lymph-nodes in patients with prostate cancer. J Urol 170:1798–1803
11. Ross PL, Scardino PT, Kattan MW (2001) A catalog of prostate cancer nomograms. J Urol 165:1562–1568
12. Burkhard FC, Bader P, Schneider E, Markwalder R, Studer UE (2002) Reliability of preoperative values to determine the need for lymphadenectomy in patients with prostate cancer and meticulous lymph-node dissection. Eur Urol 42:84–92
13. Kondylis FI, Moriarty RP, Bostwick D, Schellhammer PF (2003) Prostate cancer grade assignment: the effect of chronological, interpretive and translational bias. J Urol 170:1189–1193
14. Gil-Vernet JM (1996) Prostate cancer: anatomical and surgical considerations. Br J Urol 78:161–168
15. Raghavaiah NV, Jordan WP Jr (1979) Prostatic lymphography. J Urol 121:178–181
16. Schuessler WW, Pharand D, Vancaillie TG (1993) Laparoscopic standard pelvic node dissection for carcinoma of the prostate: is it accurate? J Urol 150:898–901
17. Bader P, Burkhard FC, Markwalder R, Studer UE (2002) Is limited lymph-node dissection an adequate staging procedure for prostate cancer? J Urol 168:514–518
18. McDowell GC 2nd, Johnson JW, Tenney DM, Johnson DE (1990) Pelvic lymphadenectomy for staging localised prostate cancer. Indication, complication and results in 217 cases. Urology 35:476–482
19. Clark T, Parekh DJ, Cookson MS, et al (2003) Randomised prospective evaluation of extended versus limited lymph-node dissection in patients with clinically localised prostate cancer. J Urol 169:145–148
20. Weingärtner K, Ramaswamy A, Bittinger A, Gerharz EW, Voge D, Riedmiller H (1996) Anatomical basis for pelvic lymphadenectomy in prostate cancer: results of an autopsy study and implications for the clinic. J Urol 156:1969–1971
21. Herrell DS, Trachtenberg J, Theodorescu D (1997) Staging pelvic lymphadenectomy for localised carcinoma of the prostate: a comparison of 3 surgical techniques. J Urol 157:1337–1339
22. Golimbu M, Morales P, Al-Askari S, Brown J (1979) Extended pelvic lymphadenectomy for prostatic cancer. J Urol 121:617–620

23. Heidenreich A, Varga Z, Knobloch RV (2002) Extended pelvic lymphadenectomy in patients undergoing radical prostatectomy: high incidence of lymph-node metastasis. J Urol 167:1681–1686

24. Allaf ME, Palapattu GS, Trock BJ, Carter HB, Walsh PC (2004) Anatomical extent of lymph-node dissection: impact on men with clinically localised prostate cancer. J Urol 172:1840–1844

25. Stone NN, Stock RG, Unger P (1997) Laparoscopic pelvic lymph-node dissection for prostate cancer: comparison of the extended and modified techniques. J Urol 158:1891–1894

26. Parkin J, Keeley FX Jr, Timoney AG (2002) Laparoscopic lymph-node sampling in locally advanced prostate cancer. BJU Int 89:14–18

27. Shackley DC, Irving SO, Brough WA, O'Reilly PH (1999) Staging laparoscopic pelvic lymphadenectomy in prostate cancer. BJU Int 83:260–264

28. Lezin SM, Cherrie R, Cattolica EV (1997) Comparison of laparoscopic and minilaparotomy pelvic lymphadenectomy for prostate cancer staging in a community practice. Urology 49:60–64

29. [No authors listed] (1998) Axillary dissection. The steering committee on clinical practice guidelines for the care and treatment of breast cancer. Canadian Association of Radiation Oncologists. CMAJ 158 [Suppl 3]: S22–26

30. Bonencamp JJ, Hermans J, Sasako M, et al (1999) Extended lymph-node dissection for gastric cancer. NEJM 340:908–914

31. Epstein JI, Oesterling JE, Eggleston JC, Walsh PC (1986) Frozen section detection of lymph-node metastases in prostatic carcinoma: accuracy in grossly uninvolved pelvic lymphadenectomy specimens. J Urol 136:1234–1237

32. Young MPA, Kirby RS, O'Donoghue EPN, Parkinson MC (1999) Accuracy and cost of intraoperative lymph-node frozen sections at radical prostatectomy. J Clin Pathol 52:925–927

33. Beissner RS, Stricker JB, Speights VO, Coffield KS, Spiekerman AM, Riggs M (2002) Frozen section diagnosis of metastatic prostate adenocarcinoma in pelvic lymphadenectomy compared with nomogram prediction of metastasis. Urology 59:721–725

34. Winstanley AM, Sandison A, Bott SRJ, Dogan A, Parkinson MC (2002) Incidental findings in pelvic lymph-nodes at radical prostatectomy. J Clin Pathol 55:623–626

35. Scott KW, Grace RH (1989) Detection of lymph-node metastases in colorectal carcinoma before and after fat clearance. Br J Surg 76:1165–1167

36. Goldstein NS (2002) Lymph-node recoveries from 2427 pT3 colorectal resection specimens spanning 45 years: recommendations for a minimum number of recovered lymph-nodes based on predictive probabilities. Am J Surg Pathol 26:179–189

37. Barth PJ, Gerharz EW, Ramaswamy A, Riedmiller H (1999) The influence of lymph-node counts on the detection of pelvic lymph-node metastasis in prostate cancer. Pathol Res Pract 195:633–636

38. Verrill C, Carr NJ, Wilkinson-Smith E, Seel EH (2004) Histopathological assessment of lymph-nodes in colorectal carcinoma: does triple levelling detect significantly more metastases? J Clin Pathol 57:1165–1167

39. Wawroschek F, Wagner T, Hamm M, et al (2003) The influence of serial sections, immunohistochemistry and extension of pelvic lymph-node dissection on the lymph-node status in clinically localised prostate cancer. Eur Urol 43:132–137

40. Rukstalis DB, Gerber GS, Vogelzang NJ, Haraf DJ, Straus FH 2nd, Chodak GW (1994) Laparoscopic pelvic lymph-node dissection: a review of 103 consecutive cases. J Urol 151:670–674

41. Solberg A, Angelsen A, Bergen U, Haugen OA, Viset T, Klepp O (2003) Frequency of lymphocoele after open and laparoscopic pelvic lymph-node dissection in patients with prostate cancer. Scand J Urol Nephrol 37:218–221

42. Wawroschek F, Hamm M, Weckermann D, Vogt H, Harzmann R (2003) Lymph-node staging in clinically localised prostate cancer. Urol Int 71:129–135

43. Brenot-Rossi I, Bastide C, Garcia S, et al (2005) Limited pelvic lymphadenectomy using the sentinel lymph-node procedure in patients with localised prostate carcinoma: a pilot study. Eur J Nucl Mol Imaging 32:635–640

44. Spellman MC, Castellino RA, Ray GR, Pistenma DA, Bagshaw MA (1997) An evaluation of lymphography in localized carcinoma of the prostate. Radiology 125:637–644

45. Wallace S, Jing BS, Zornoza J (1977) Lymphangiography in the determination of the extent of metastatic carcinoma: the potential value of percutaneous lymph node biopsy. Cancer 39 [Suppl 2]:706–718

46. Wolf JS Jr, Cher M, Dall'Era M, Presti JC Jr, Hricak H, Carroll PR (1995) Prostate cancer: the use and accuracy of cross sectional imaging and fine needle aspiration cytology for detection of pelvic lymph-node metastases before radical prostatectomy. J Urol 153 [Suppl 3S]: 993–999

47. Borley NC, Fabrin K, Sriprasad S, Mondani N et al. (2003) Laparoscopic pelvic lymph-node dissection allows significantly more accurate staging on "high risk" prostate cancer compared to MRI or CT. Scand J Urol Nephrology 37:382–386

48. Ponsky LE, Cherullo EE, Starkey R, Nelson D, Neumann D, Zippe CD (2002) Evaluation of pre-operative ProstaScint scans in the prediction of nodal disease. Prostate Cancer Prostatic Dis 5:132–135

49. Schoder H, Larson SM (2004) Positron emission tomography for prostate, bladder and renal cancer. Semin Nucl Med 34:274–292

50. de Jong IJ, Pruim J, Elsinga PH, Vaalburg W, Mensink HJ (2003) Preoperative staging of pelvic lymph-node in prostate cancer by 11C-choline PET. J Nucl Med 44:331–335

51. Harisinghani MG, Barentsz J, Hahn PF, Deserno WM et al. (2003) Nonivasive detection of clinically occult lymph-node metastases in prostate cancer. N Engl Med J 348:2491–2499

Technique of Endoscopic Extraperitoneal Radical Prostatectomy – Step by Step

7

Jens-Uwe Stolzenburg · Robert Rabenalt · Minh Do · Evangelos Liatsikos

Contents

In the present chapter we will go through the technique of EERPE. For didactic reasons we will present every single step of the operation with a drawing and a corresponding endoscopic image. Both conventional (wide excision) and intrafascial nerve-sparing procedures will be presented step by step. The authors gratefully acknowledge the assistance of Mr. Jens Mondry in preparing the computer imagings and Mr. Gottfried Müller in preparing the black and white figures (hand drawings).

7.1 Operative Set-up and Trocar Placement

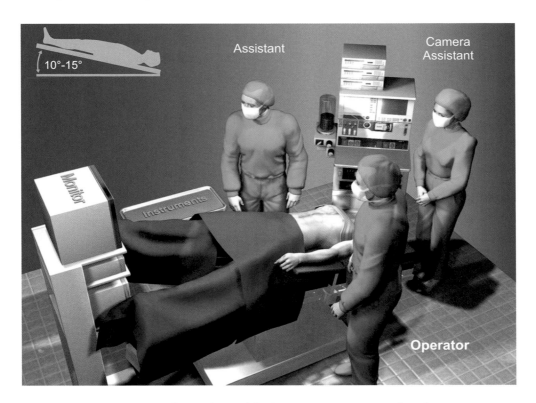

The patient is placed in a classical Trendelenburg position, or in a dorsal supine position with legs slightly apart. With increasing experience we realised that there was no need for an extreme Trendelenburg position and that 10° head-down tilt was sufficient for performing the procedure, since the bowel did not interfere with this procedure. In addition, even long operating times in difficult cases can be managed without cardiopulmonary limitations. We prefer a single video monitor at the foot end so that the surgeon and the assistant can work without any problem of mirror imaging. The monitor is placed at the bottom of the operating table as close as possible to the surgeon's eye level. The surgeon stands to the left of the patient with an assistant opposite. The camera holder stands behind the head of the patient. The scrub nurse can also act as camera holder because the procedure requires only few instruments.

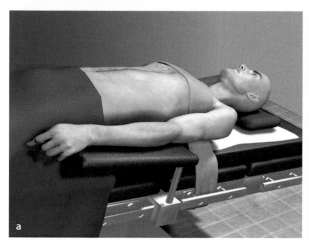
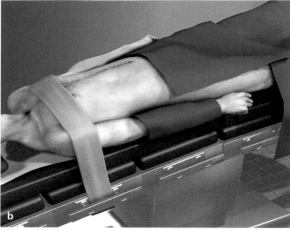

The patient is draped on the table with a chest belt. Care should be taken not to exert too much tension. The belt serves only to stabilise the patient. The right arm is draped adherent to the patient's body, and the left arm is accessible by the anaesthesiologist. Two intravenous peripheral lines are placed in the left arm. Extensions should be placed by the anaesthesiologist so access can be ascertained after covering the head of the patient. There is no need for central lines.

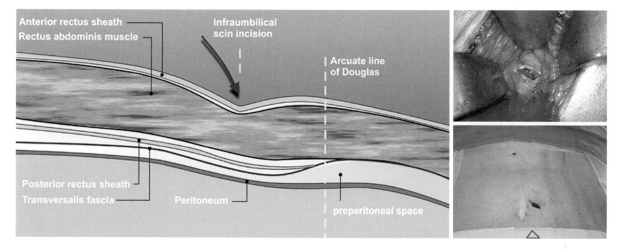

The first step of the procedure is to create a preperitoneal space and the placement of the first trocar. A 12- to 15-mm incision is made 1 cm below and lateral to the umbilicus (right paraumbilical incision) (*lower right*). We prefer not to make the incision in the midline, avoiding the linea alba adhesions. The *left image* shows the layers of the abdominal wall. After the right infraumbilical incision, a blunt dissection is performed down to the anterior rectus sheath. The anterior rectus sheath is slightly horizontally incised (*upper right*), and this opening is enlarged by blunt dissection (to avoid any bleeding) with the help of scissors. Specially designed hooks used by the assistant are very helpful (see Chap. 3.1). As soon as the horizontal fascial incision is performed the longitudinal muscle fibres of the rectus muscle become visible.

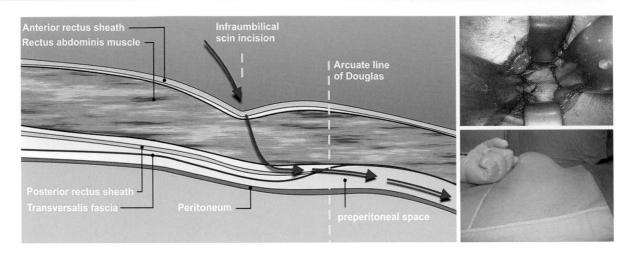

7

Only blunt dissection is used to separate the muscle fibres of the rectus muscle. Again the specially designed hooks are very helpful. The assistant has to change the direction of the hook retraction from horizontal to vertical. The posterior rectus fascia is then exposed (*upper right*). Be aware that the thickness of the muscle differs from patient to patient. In very obese patients longer hooks are needed.

The space between the rectus muscle and the posterior rectus sheath is bluntly developed by finger dissection in the direction of the preperitoneal space (*lower right*). Be careful with epigastric vessels on the right side. Vigorous dissection could injure them. Extensive blunt finger dissection is not needed.

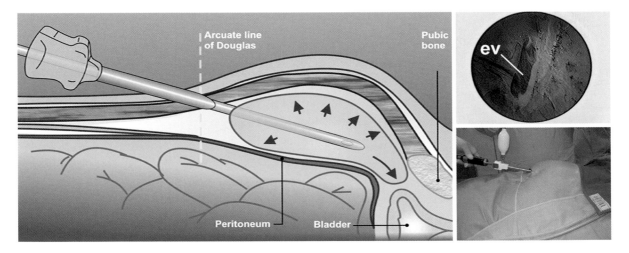

A balloon trocar is introduced superior to the posterior rectus sheath and insufflated under direct visual control. The posterior rectus sheath is absent inferior to the arcuate line. That is why the balloon dilation creates the preperitoneal space. The epigastric vessels are first seen ventrally compressed through the balloon (upper right). The epigastric vessels and the pubic arch are the main landmarks during balloon dilation. The pubic arch becomes visible towards the end of the dissection.

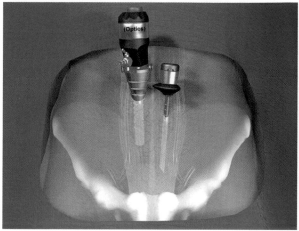
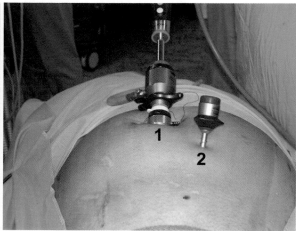

The balloon trocar is removed and stay sutures are then placed at either end of the anterior rectus sheath incision. An optical trocar (Hassan type) is introduced and fixed (trocar number 1). After insufflation with CO_2 (12 mmHg), a 5-mm trocar (trocar number 2) is positioned 2 fingertips left, lateral to the midline (one-third of the way from the umbilicus to the pubic arch).

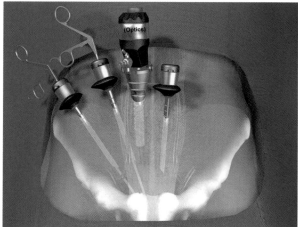
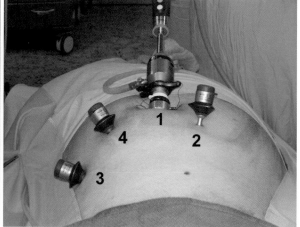

A 5-mm trocar (trocar number 3) is then positioned two fingers medial to the right anterior superior iliac spine (in the line from the spine to the umbilicus). Another 5-mm trocar (trocar number 4) is placed in the right pararectal line (on the same theoretical line from the spine to the umbilicus) taking care to avoid injury of the epigastric vessels.

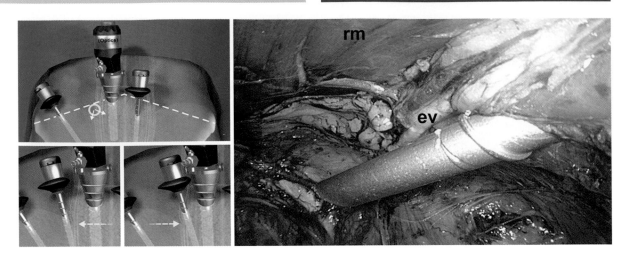

7

Injury to the epigastric vessels can be caused during insertion of the fourth trocar (pararectal line, right iliac fossa). For this reason this is the most dangerous trocar for bleeding. Injury to the epigastric vessels can be avoided by careful inspection of the abdominal wall via the laparoscope before trocar insertion. The fourth trocar position has to be varied medially or laterally (see *arrows*) aiming to avoid epigastric vessel injury. Another way to reduce the risk of injury is to use a Versastep trocar.

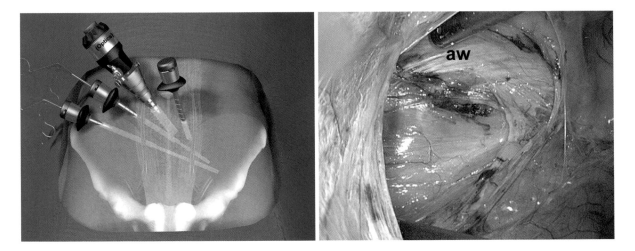

Operating bimanually through trocars number 3 and 4, dissection is continued bluntly to the left preperitoneal space. Follow the pubic arch from right to left and then identify the iliac vessels and spermatic cord. Go ventrally and dissect underneath the epigastric vessels to the left side. Most dissection can be performed bluntly. If the assistant is not experienced, the surgeon should then change his position and move to the right side of the patient for this step.

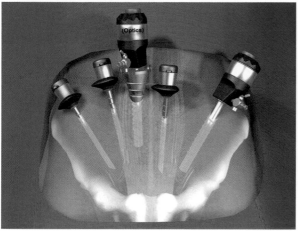
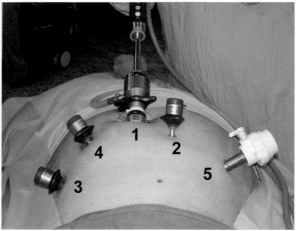

The final 12-mm trocar is placed approximately three finger breaths medial to the left anterior superior iliac spine (on a hypothetical line from the spine to the umbilicus). Avoid placement too distally or too close to the iliac spine, because this can cause problems during apical dissection and anastomosis. This is the trocar through which all the lymph nodes are extracted. Furthermore, the needles are inserted and extracted through this trocar.

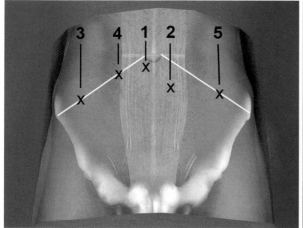
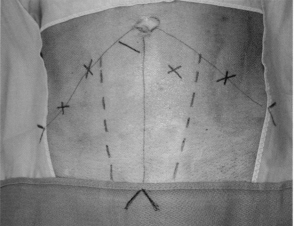

This figure summarises the position of all trocars. The imaginary lines drawn in the pictures are helpful for orientation (from umbilicus to anterior superior iliac spine – continuous lines; pararectal line – interrupted lines). The numbers give the sequence of trocar placement.

7

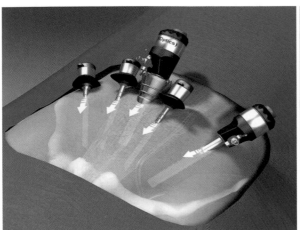
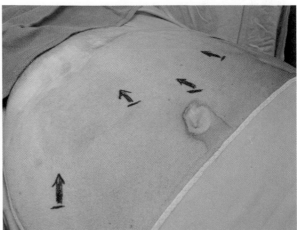

In extremely obese or very tall patients, all trocars should be placed 1–3 cm caudally, depending on the size of the patient, for optimal access to the retropubic space. The principles of trocar placement are the same. In extremely obese patients a 10+5° head-down position is recommended.

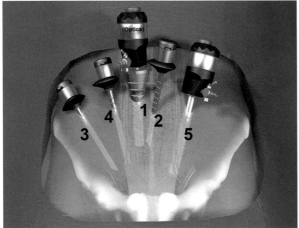
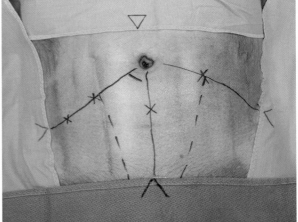

Trocar positioning in a patient with previous left inguinal hernia repair with mesh placement. The initial camera port placement and balloon insufflation of the extraperitoneal space are achieved in the same way as previously described. The subsequent steps are modified. A second 5-mm trocar is placed directly in the midline one-third of the way from the umbilicus to the pubic symphysis. This is deliberately more medial than usual. Working with grasping forceps through the second trocar, the extraperitoneal space is carefully developed laterally to the right. The third and fourth trocars are placed in the usual positions. A space for safe placement of the fifth trocar (12 mm) in the left pararectal line is created without disrupting the adhesions in the left inguinal region.

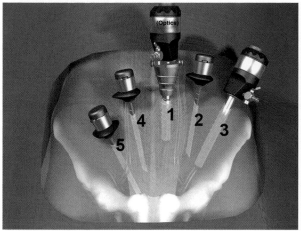
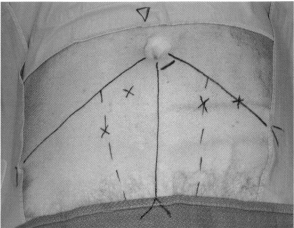

Trocar positioning in a patient with previous right inguinal hernia repair with mesh placement. In contrast to the classical technique, the first skin incision is made in the left paraumbilical region. The second trocar (5 mm) is placed in the left pararectal line, and the creation of the extraperitoneal space is continued with forceps through this trocar. When the peritoneum has been completely dissected free from the posterior aspect of the left rectus muscle, a third trocar (12 mm) is placed approximately two finger breadths medial to the left anterior superior iliac spine. Because of the anticipated fibrosis, placement of the usual extreme right lateral trocar is not attempted. There is consequently no extensive dissection necessary in the right inguinal region. Instead, a fourth trocar (5 mm) is placed at the intersection between the pararectal line and the imaginary line between the anterior superior iliac spine and the umbilicus. The fifth trocar is placed in the pararectal line 3–4 cm above the symphysis.

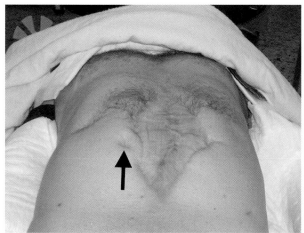
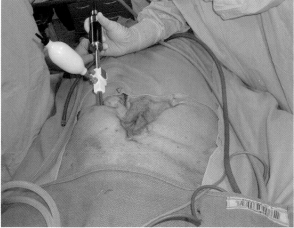

This patient had previous abdominal surgery for colon carcinoma. He developed peritonitis and three reinterventions were performed. The insertion of a mesh was deemed necessary to close the fascias and wound. Note the extensive scar on the mid and lower abdomen with a lateral dislocation of the umbilicus (*arrow*). The creation of the preperitoneal space and the placement of the first trocar starts "classically" (right infraumbilical incision, visualisation of the posterior rectus sheath, finger and balloon dissection).

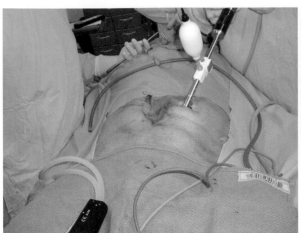
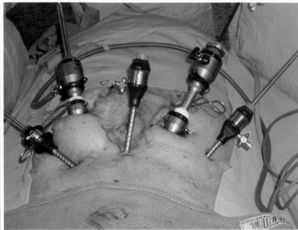

7

The initial trocar had to be placed laterally due to the extensive scar formation, and thus the retroperitoneal space could not be completely created. Therefore, a second balloon dilation of the retroperitoneal space is performed from the left side. Final trocar placement is different to the typical EERPE. The number of trocars are the same (three 5 mm, two 10 mm), but we use two Hassan trocars instead of one. The position of the trocars is changed according to the available space. In general, flexibility of trocar sites is necessary when dealing with difficult cases and should not be a problem for an experienced surgeon.

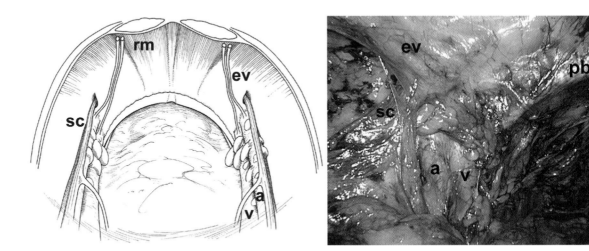

This figure shows the landmarks of the preperitoneal space after trocar placement: ventrally the rectus muscle; lateral to the rectus muscle, the inferior epigastric vessels converging on the external iliac vessels, which are located craniolaterally to the pubic arch and covered by the lymph nodes. The spermatic cord containing the vas runs into the inguinal ring.

7.2 Pelvic Lymph Node Dissection

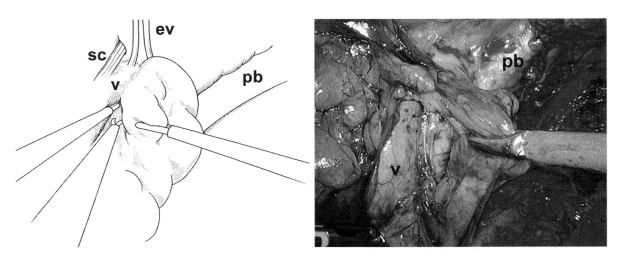

The lymphadenectomy starts on the left side. For orientation find the junction of the epigastric and iliac vessels. The assistant has to retract on the lymph node and the surgeon dissects between the lymph node (and fatty tissue) and the iliac vessels. The lymph vessels are located, clipped and cut with the aid of the SonoSurg device. If you encounter problems identifying the lymph node, search for the iliac artery (pulsation) and start dissection from there.

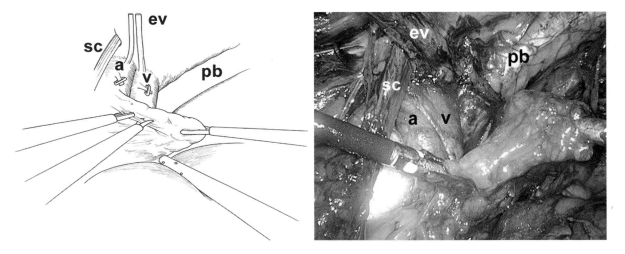

The external iliac artery and vein are then meticulously cleaned from their surrounding lymphatic tissue. All lymphatic vessels are carefully clipped and dissected with the SonoSurg. The assistant retracts the lymphatic tissue craniolaterally to his side, with his right instrument. The peritoneum is pushed cranially by the assistant's left instrument (suction tube).

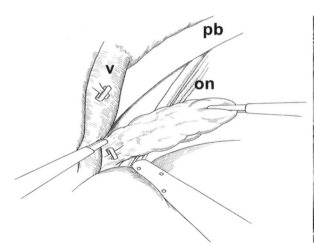

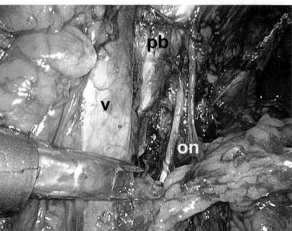

7

The next step of the lymphadenectomy is the dissection of the lymphatic tissue from the obturator fossa. The nerve is freed from caudal to cranial. Care should be taken not to injure the accompanying artery and vein. In the case of bleeding the vessels should be clipped, and extensive coagulation should be avoided (thermal injury of the obturator nerve). The dissection within the cranial end of the fossa is often cumbersome. The role of the assistant is crucial at this point.

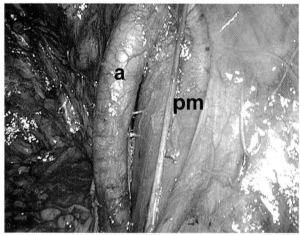

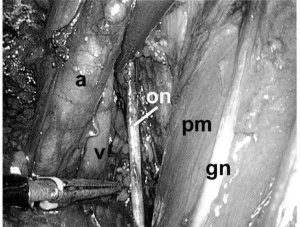

The *left image* shows the completely cleaned external iliac artery and its adjacent psoas muscle and genito-femoralis nerve (lateral border for the lymphadenectomy). The *right image* shows the complete lymphatic dissection after cleaning the posterior aspect of the external iliac artery and vein. The vessels are retracted medially and the entire obturator fossa is thus completely freed from its lymphatic tissue.

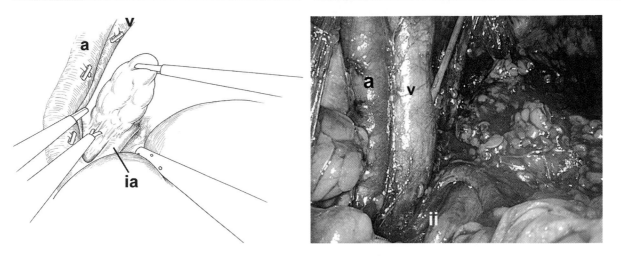

Starting from the external iliac artery the dissection is continued in a caudo-cranial direction. The junction of the internal iliac with the external iliac artery is the upper end of the lymph node dissection (standard lymphadenectomy). Care should be taken to avoid ureteral injury. Extended lymphadenectomy including the common iliac and the entire internal iliac artery is extremely difficult or impossible with extraperitoneal access. The same operative steps are performed on the right side. In most steps the surgeon has to apply traction on the lymphatic tissue.

7.3 "Wide Excision" EERPE

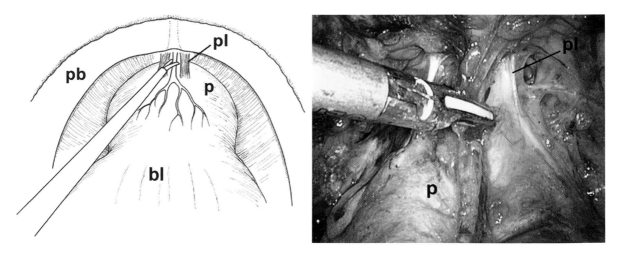

The operation is now continued by a dissection of the whole Retzius space from the symphysis down to the apex of the prostate. Take care to drain the bladder completely. The fatty and areolar tissue is swept gently from the anterior surface of the bladder neck, from the anterior surface of the prostate and the endopelvic fascia. Use of the bipolar forceps is advised. The superficial branch of the dorsal vein has to be exposed, coagulated and cut with the aid of the SonoSurg device.

7

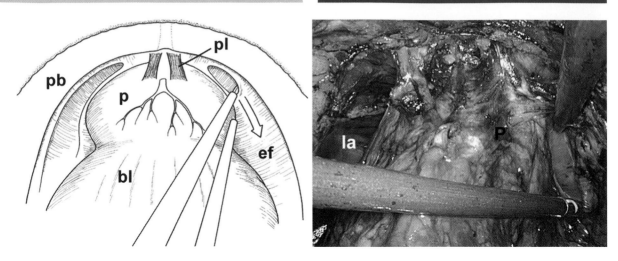

The endopelvic fascia is incised on both sides. Initial incision is performed as shown in the picture. At this level the distinction between the lateral side of the prostate and the endopelvic fascia covering the levator ani muscle is evident. Blunt dissection is performed proximally towards the bladder and towards the apex. Sharp dissection ,may be necessary toward the apex in the case of adhesions. The prostate is retracted medially by the assistant to free any fibres of the levator ani that remain attached to the prostate.

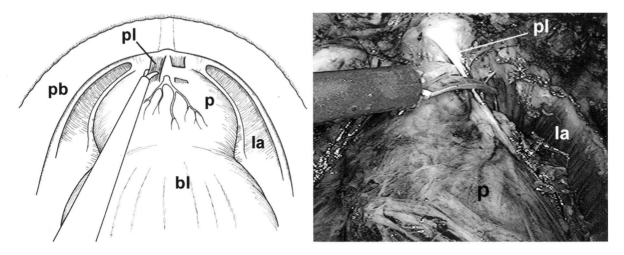

Both puboprostatic ligaments are fully dissected with cold scissors. The Santorini venous plexus is situated directly under the ligaments. Take care not to cut too deep. The ligaments are avascular and no bleeding is expected. The dissection of the ligaments can also be performed with the aid of the SonoSurg device.

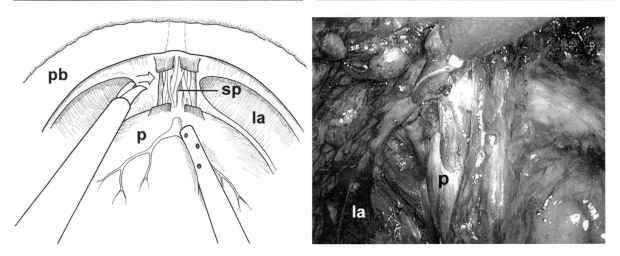

Once the ligaments are completely dissected, the apex of the prostate is more clearly seen. The remaining segments of the endopelvic fascia, and any possible adhesions, are dissected. Sometimes, venous tributaries pass from the levator ani muscle to the prostate just lateral to the puboprostatic ligament. Caution should be made to coagulate with bipolar forceps or dissect with the SonoSurg device.

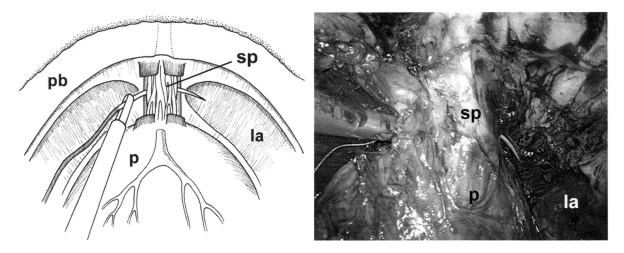

The prostate is now retracted caudally by the assistant for good access to the Santorini plexus and adequate needle manoeuvrability. The Santorini plexus is ligated with 2–0 Polysorb (GS-22 needle, slightly straightened) by selective passage of the needle underneath the plexus from left to right. If the initial ligation is not safe, do not hesitate to stitch a second time with the same needle. When a stitch is considered to be positioned too deep towards the urethra (very seldom), the urethral catheter should be moved, ruling out its entrapment by the suture. The dorsal venous plexus is not divided following ligation. It is divided at the end of the dissection of the prostate to avoid unnecessary bleeding.

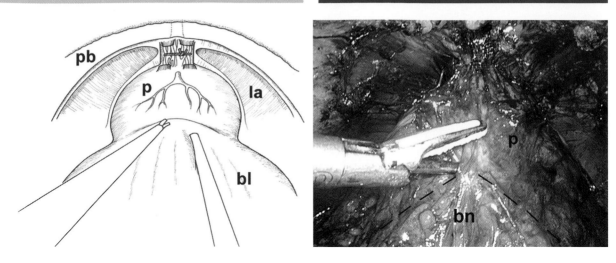

The bladder neck can be identified after removal of all the prevesical fatty tissue. It overlaps the prostate in the shape of a triangle (see *interrupted lines*). The urethral catheter balloon is deflated before beginning the dissection. The dissection starts at a 12 o' clock position at the tip of this triangle. Palpation with the forceps helps to identify the border between the mobile bladder neck and the solid prostate in difficult cases. When the border between prostate and bladder is not evident, repeated traction on the catheter helps to identify the limit between the mobile bladder neck and the solid prostate. It is clear that the balloon of the urethral catheter must be inflated for this manoeuvre.

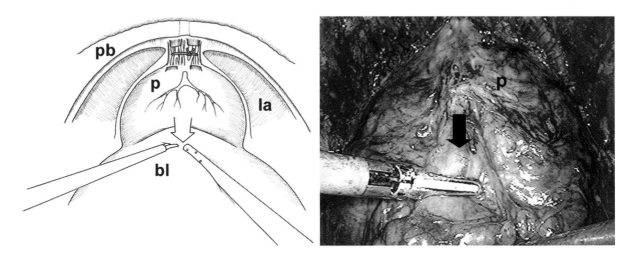

When the appropriate plane between the prostate and bladder is not clearly seen, the dissection of the bladder neck should be performed more proximally (toward the bladder – *arrow*), thus avoiding intrusion within the prostatic tissue. It is always better to reconstruct a wider bladder neck than to risk a positive margin at the bladder neck. Bladder neck preservation is technically demanding.

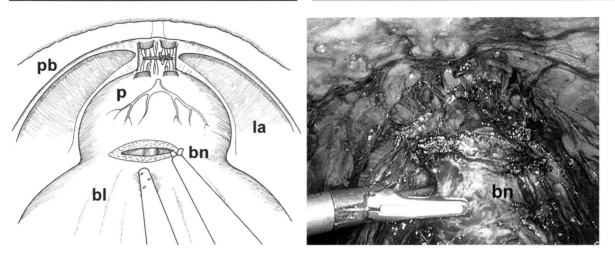

A transverse incision is made from the 10 o' clock to the 2 o' clock position with the SonoSurg device, and the bladder neck is developed with blunt and sharp dissection. The assistant has to push the bladder dorsally with the aid of the suction.

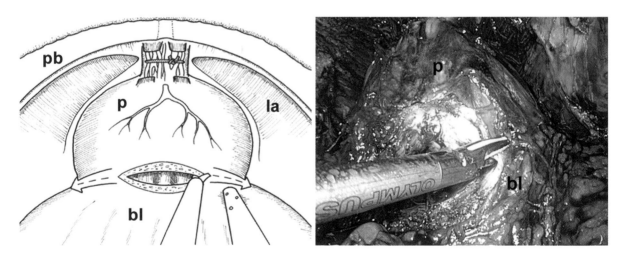

The dissection is now continued to the lateral direction in the plane between bladder neck and prostate. Note that the bladder neck is not fully dissected. We only dissect the superficial layers, facilitating the sparing of the bladder neck. The bipolar forceps is used to control minor vessels. Once again, the assistant pushes the bladder dorsally with his instruments.

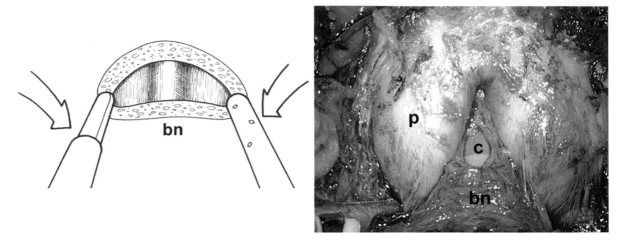

7

Blunt dissection is then performed and the longitudinal musculature of the bladder neck is developed. The surgeon and the assistant push the basis of the developed bladder neck dorsally for better visualisation of the bladder neck. The surgeon then develops the longitudinal musculature of the bladder neck. In bladder neck-sparing procedures this step must be performed very meticulously. Once the longitudinal musculature of the bladder neck is fully developed, the catheter morphology is starting to be evident. The circumference of the urethra is developed anterolaterally and an incision is made at the 12 o'clock position.

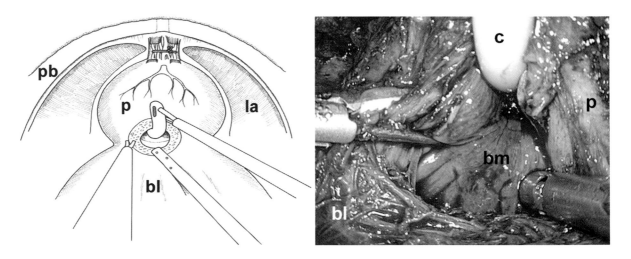

When the bladder is incised more proximally, as shown in the previous figure on page 80, preservation of the bladder neck is not feasible. The bladder neck is incised and the bladder mucosa becomes clearly visible. The deflated balloon catheter is pulled up into the retropubic space by the assistant under continuous tension.

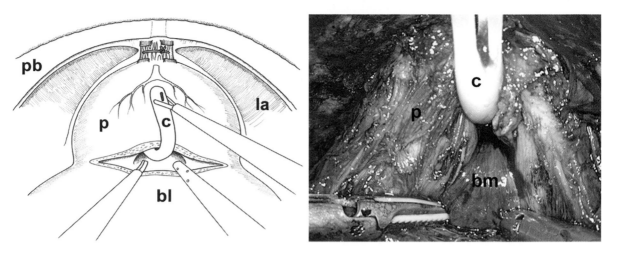

In the bladder neck-sparing technique, as soon as the urethra is incised at the 12 o'clock position the catheter is pulled by the assistant towards the symphysis. Note that you should exert traction to the catheter with a clamp at the level of the urethral meatus. The dissection is now continued to the lateral direction in the plane between bladder neck and prostate. The dissection is performed with the help of the SonoSurg device. The magnification of the laparoscope helps to identify the mucosa of the bladder. The mucosa is the key structure that leads our dissection. If you get lost during dissection, go back to the midline, identify the bladder neck mucosa and start again from there.

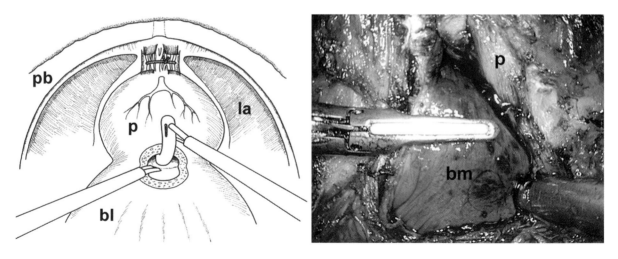

Before starting the posterior bladder neck dissection make sure that the natural groove between bladder mucosa and prostate in the dorsal direction can be identified. Transection of the posterior bladder neck is performed with the SonoSurg device. It is of outmost importance that the assistant exerts traction on the catheter so the posterior bladder neck is ideally exposed.

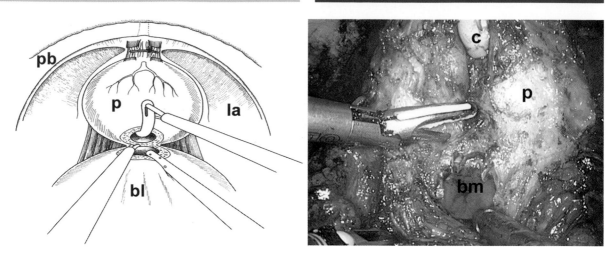

7

It is easier to dissect the posterior bladder neck when you expand the dissection laterally, freeing the prostate from the bladder. Note that the dissection needs to follow a perpendicular plane to ascertain access to the seminal vesicles. It is important to avoid oblique dissection because you will end up dissecting within the prostate.

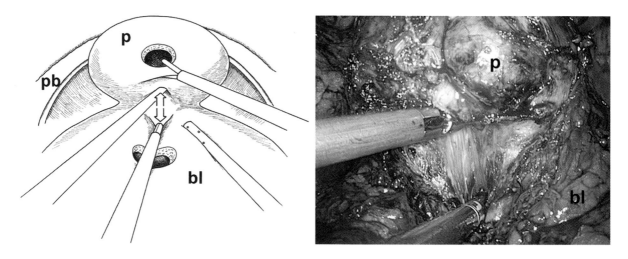

The bladder neck is first completely divided between the 5 and 7 o'clock positions. Then the surgeon bluntly enlarges this space with his instruments as shown in the figure. This blunt dissection should be performed without any particular problems. If dissection is not feasible, consider that you may not be in the correct plane of dissection. The assistant should release the catheter tip, grasp the posterior part of the prostate and pull it under tension cranially. Then the surgeon must go back to midline and visualise the bladder neck and start dissection again. The most common mistake is to dissect too obliquely and end up within the prostate.

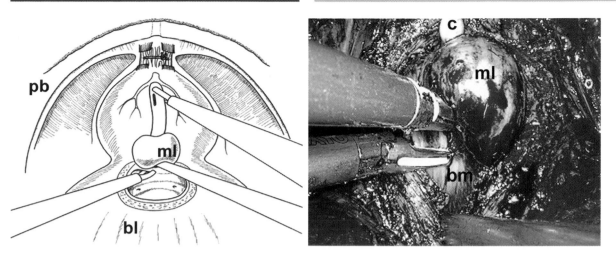

In the case of a middle lobe the fold between the middle lobe and the bladder mucosa is usually clearly visible. The orifices can be very close to the plane of dissection. In the case of a large middle lobe, identify the orifices before dissecting the posterior bladder neck. For beginners we recommend insertion of double pigtail catheters prior to surgery.

Under normal conditions, the ureteral orifices are far away from the bladder neck incision. When a transurethral prostatectomy has been previously performed the ureteral orifices are retracted towards the bladder neck. Preoperative insertion of double pigtail ureteral catheters is necessary to identify the orifices and avoid their injury.

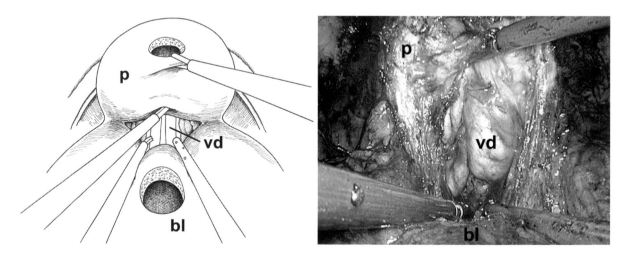

The end point of the posterior bladder neck dissection is the identification of the anatomical landmarks of the ampullary portions of the seminal vesicles. When these structures are identified the posterior bladder neck dissection is extended laterally in both directions. Always check the bladder mucosa before the extensive lateral dissection to avoid bladder injury.

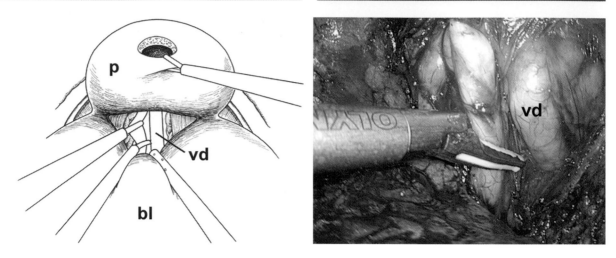

7

The left vas is grasped by the surgeon and developed. The vas should not be dissected directly at the level of the prostate. It should be dissected distally towards the bladder. This facilitates later access to the seminal vesicles. It is important that the assistant pushes the bladder down to get better access to the vas.

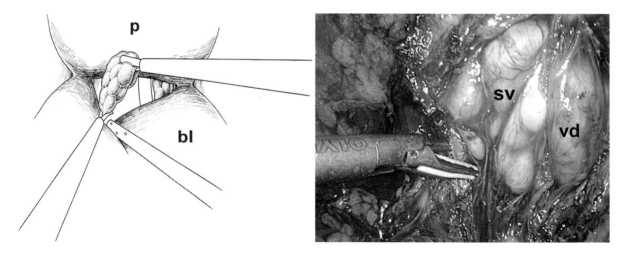

The seminal vesicles can be identified in a slightly lateral direction. The assistant retracts the seminal vesicle laterally and cranially with the forceps on his right hand, and with the suction on his left hand he pushes the bladder down. This provides good visualisation of the left seminal vesicle. The surgeon can now begin dissecting the seminal vesicle step by step from its surrounding structures. The magnification of the laparoscope helps to reveal the supplying arteries of the seminal vesicles. These arteries have to be dissected with the help of the SonoSurg device to avoid any bleeding.

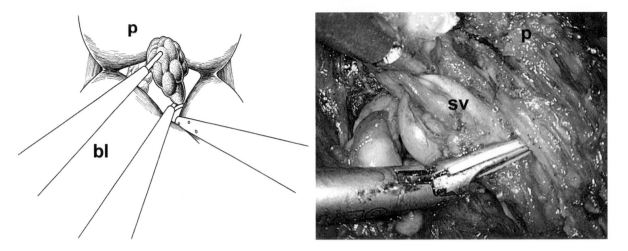

On the right side the surgeon grasps the seminal vesicle and applies tension contralaterally and cranially with the forceps on his left hand. With the SonoSurg device on his right hand he performs the complete dissection of the seminal vesicle. Blunt dissection can be performed when possible. When bleeding is encountered bipolar cautery is used.

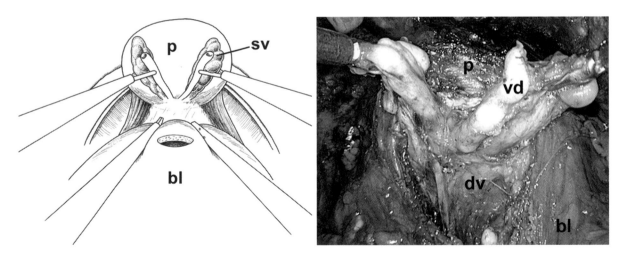

After dissection of the seminal vesicles the assistant holds the right ampulla and the right seminal vesicle, the surgeon the left ampulla and the left seminal vesicle in a craniolateral direction. With this manoeuvre a "window" is developed which reaches from the dorsal aspect of the prostate to the prostatic pedicles. Between these structures the posterior layer of Denonvilliers' fascia is clearly seen.

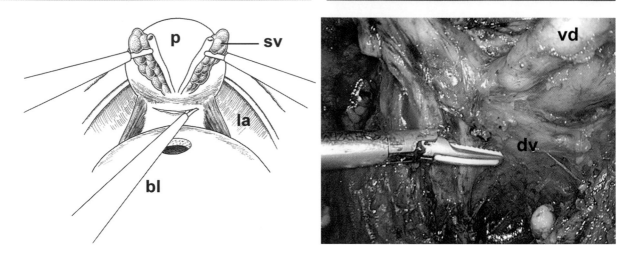

7

A horizontal incision is performed on the posterior layer of Denonvilliers' fascia. If you have problems identifying the correct plane, feel the solid structure of the prostate and stay close to its posterior surface.

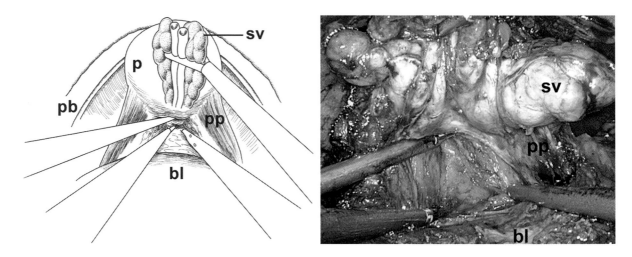

After incision of Denonvilliers' fascia the prerectal fatty tissue (yellow in colour) is visualised. The dissection is continued as far as possible towards the apex of the prostate in the midline. The rectum is thus pushed away from the plane of dissection. Blunt dissection is performed in two manners: first cranio-caudally along the sulcus of the prostate, and then medio-laterally in the direction of the prostatic pedicles. The visualisation of the posterior plane of the prostate ascertains a safe plane of dissection, especially during later prostatic pedicle dissection.

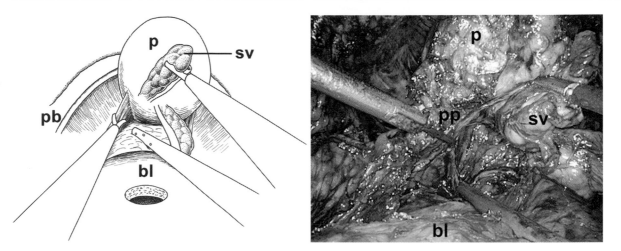

The next manoeuvre is designed to place the prostatic pedicles in tension. To accomplish this, the assistant again elevates the left seminal vesicle in a contralateral cranial direction out of the pelvis. In that way, the left prostate pedicle can easily be identified as a cord structure. The pedicle and the neurovascular bundle are then dissected with the aid of the SonoSurg device (surgeon's left hand). We suggest the use of the "slower" energy option of the SonoSurg for better haemostasis. If there is residual bleeding use bipolar forceps or clips.

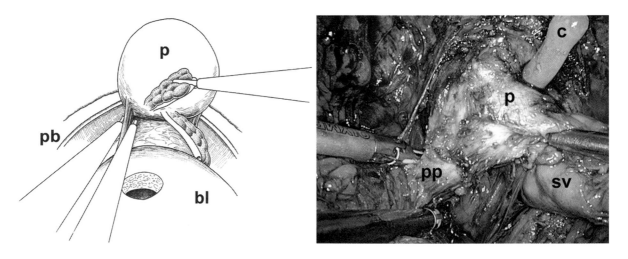

Tip: If you lose the plane of dissection go back to the bladder neck, get the assistant to pull more on the prostate, push the rectum down in the midline with the forceps in your right hand, and use the instrument in your left hand lateral to the pedicle as shown in this figure. By pushing both instruments down and converging to the midline you should find the right plane.

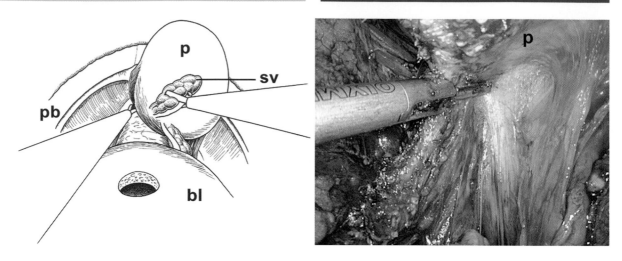

This dissection is performed to a point just cephalad to the apex and the urethra. When the assistant continues to maintain the traction on the base of the seminal vesicle, the prostate is pulled more and more out of the pelvis.

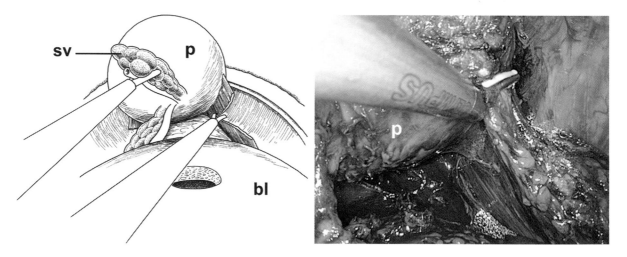

The same manoeuvre is performed on the right side. The surgeon exerts the traction on the seminal vesicle with the forceps in his left hand, and he performs the dissection with the SonoSurg device in his right hand. The assistant helps by pushing the bladder and rectum out of the working field.

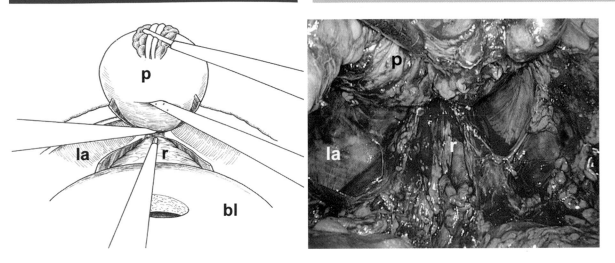

Final midline attachments of the posterior surface of the prostate to the rectum should be bluntly detached whenever possible (in most cases). In that way, the prostate is completely mobilised anteriorly, laterally and posteriorly.

7.4 Nerve-sparing EERPE

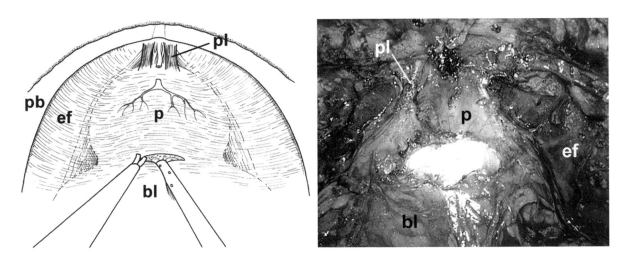

The anterior surface of the bladder neck and prostate and the endopelvic fascia are exposed and the fatty tissue overlying these structures is gently swept away. The superficial branch of the deep dorsal vein complex is fulgurated with bipolar forceps and divided. The endopelvic fascia is not incised as performed in our previously described technique, and the Santorini plexus is not ligated at the beginning of the procedure. The superficial fascia overlaying the bladder neck is then identified and dissection is initiated at the 10 to 2 o'clock position.

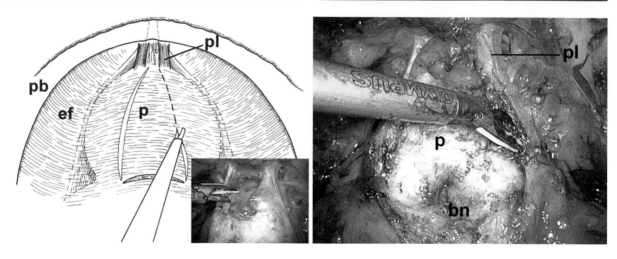

7

Starting from the bladder neck a bilateral sharp incision of the superficial fascia overlaying the prostate is performed distally toward the apex medially to the puboprostatic ligaments. The main goal is to create the landmarks where further dissection will be performed later during the procedure. This manoeuvre ascertains preservation of the puboprostatic ligaments.

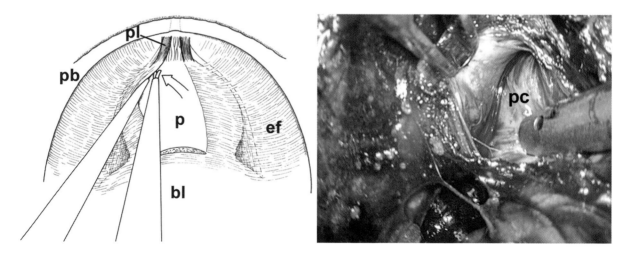

A plane is developed between the prostate and its thin overlaying fascia (periprostatic fascia). The principal goal is to develop the right plane and finally detach the prostate from its "envelopment", leaving intact the puboprostatic ligaments, the periprostatic fascia, and the endopelvic fascia as a continuous structure. The development of the plane is easier to perform towards the apex, as seen in the figure.

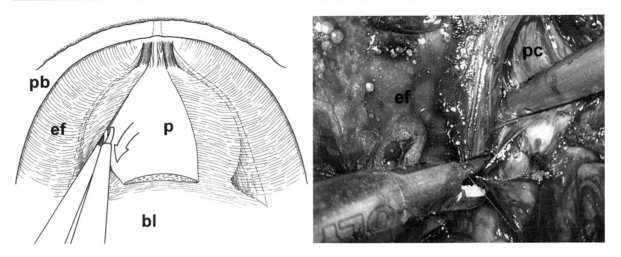

The development of the plane is then continued in an ascending fashion towards the bladder neck. When you are in the right plane you see a shiny surface upon the prostate which is easily detachable from the periprostatic fascia. Dissection and development of the plane between the prostate and the periprostatic fascia can be performed either with the aid of the SonoSurg device or by cold knife incision. When sharp incision is performed vessels should be clipped before cutting.

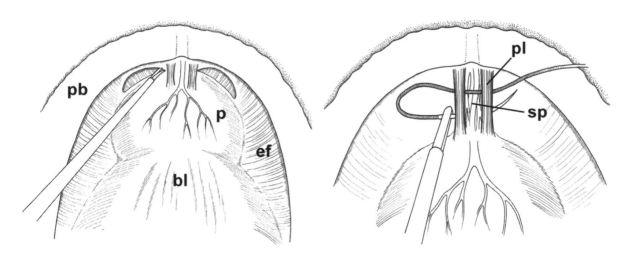

Tip: When, during the development of the plane at the apex, bleeding occurs from the Santorini venous complex you should proceed as follows. The endopelvic fascia is minimally incised, and a "window" is created, facilitating the ligation of the Santorini plexus. A 2–0 Polysorb GS-22 needle (slightly straightened to facilitate manoeuvrability) is then passed under the ligaments and over the Santorini plexus from right to left. The needle is guided from left to right in the plane below the dorsal venous complex and above the anterior urethral wall. This manoeuvre allows for plexus ligation without involvement of the puboprostatic ligaments, and should halt the bleeding.

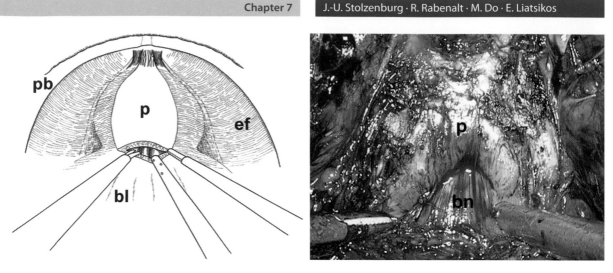

7

The next step is the bladder neck dissection. It is performed gradually, aiming to depict the longitudinal musculature of the bladder neck. See also the figures pertaining to bladder neck dissection in the wide excision technique (Sect. 7.3 above).

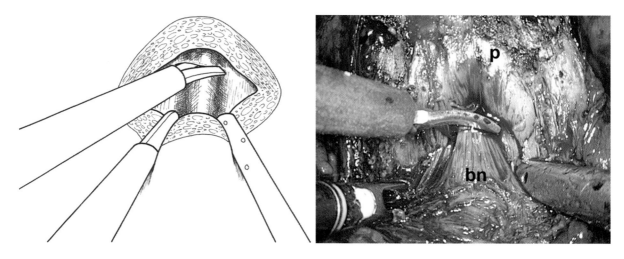

When preserving the bladder neck, the longitudinal musculature should be clearly seen and developed. This longitudinal musculature is only evident surrounding the urethra at the bladder neck. It does not exist at the lateral border between the bladder neck and the prostate. As described in Sect. 7.3, when the border between prostate and bladder is not evident, repeated traction on the catheter helps to identify the limit between the mobile bladder neck and the solid prostate.

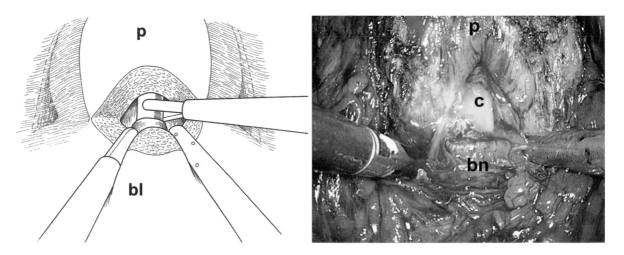

When cutting the bladder neck the assistant (with the aid of the suction) and the operator (with the aid of forceps in the right hand) have to push the bladder dorsally. In this way, the bladder neck becomes clearly visible. It is completely incised and the catheter becomes visible. The longitudinal musculature and the mucosa are two thin layers. For this reason one has to cut in minor steps. Be aware not to cut too deep. This could cause damage or even complete dissection of the catheter with dislocation of the tip of the catheter into the bladder.

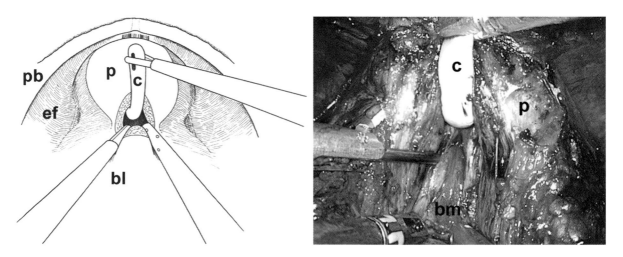

The balloon catheter is then pulled up into the retropubic space by the assistant under continuous tension. The bladder neck dissection is now continued in the lateral direction, in the plane between bladder neck and prostate, taking care not to involve the lateral tissue attachments of the prostate and bladder.

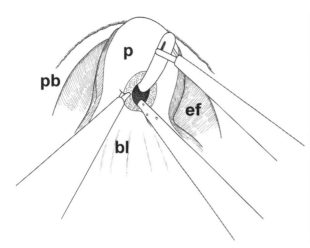

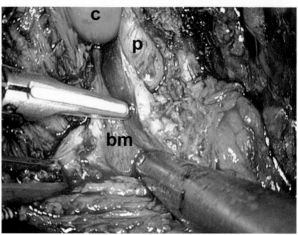

7

This figure shows the complete bladder neck dissection. The assistant has to push the bladder dorsally with the aid of the suction. The suction is directly placed into the bladder neck to visualise the mucosa. During the whole bladder neck dissection the mucosa is the key structure that leads dissection. One of the most common mistakes of beginners is the great distance of the laparoscope from the "region of interest", thus not taking advantage of the magnification of the optical system.

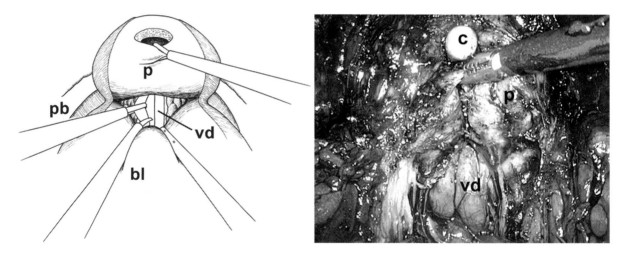

The posterior bladder neck dissection is performed as described for wide excision (Sect. 7.3). The main difference is the restricted space (window) due to the lateral attachments (fascias, nerves and vessels). The anatomical landmarks of the ampullary segments of the vas are then visualised and dissected.

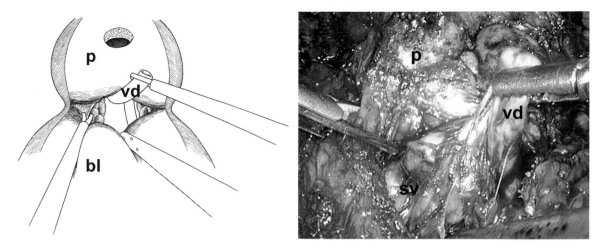

The next step of the procedure is the dissection of both vasa. Once the left vas is dissected, the assistant grasps and pulls it contralaterally towards the pubic bone. The lateral superficial attachments to the bladder are dissected. After this step the bladder neck is completely dissected in the lateral direction giving free access to the seminal vesicles. The same manoeuvre is performed on the controlateral side.

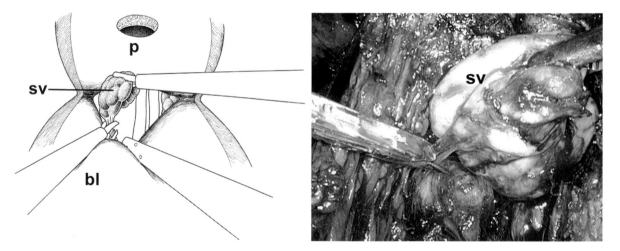

After the division of the vas the seminal vesicles are freed. Blunt and sharp dissection avoiding the use of electrocautery is recommended, especially during dissection of the tip of the seminal vesicles. The seminal vesicle is completely freed. Be careful of the arterial supply to the seminal vesicles. Such vessels should be clipped as shown in the figure, especially at the tip of the seminal vesicles. Note that too much tension on the seminal vesicles can cause damage to the nerves and injury or rupture of the arterial supply to the seminal vesicle itself. Once again, it is very important for the assistant to exert contralateral traction on the vas with the forceps in his right hand, and to push the bladder down with the instrument in his left hand.

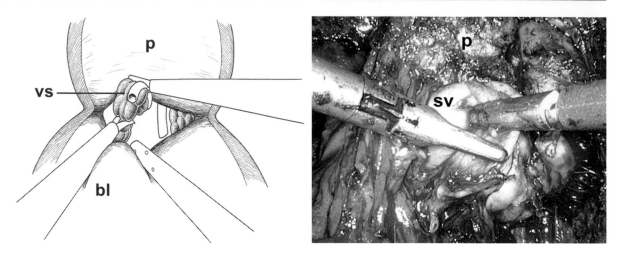

7

Some surgeons recommend not including the tips of the seminal vesicles in the surgical specimen. Their reason is the affinity of the tip of the seminal vesicles to nerve structures. They postulate that preserving the tips ascertains better potency results. We try to dissect the entire seminal vesicles whenever possible.

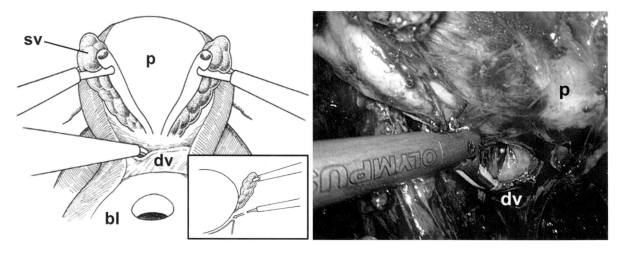

After completion of seminal vesicle dissection, the posterior layer of Denonvilliers' fascia is seen. Both the surgeon and the assistant retract the seminal vesicles in a craniolateral direction, exposing the posterior layer of Denonvilliers' fascia. In contrast to our previously described technique we do not incise the fascia. The desired plane of dissection is between Denonvilliers' fascia and the prostatic capsule, as shown in the figure.

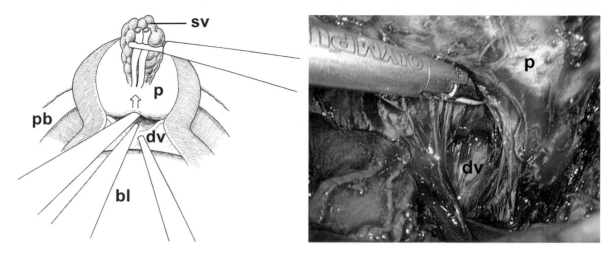

The appropriate plane is found, in most cases, by blunt dissection and by stripping down Denonvilliers' fascia from the prostatic capsule. When such dissection is not possible, a small incision can be performed to facilitate the process. In that case you will be able to see the prerectal fatty tissue. For further dissection towards the apex go back to the posterior capsular surface of the prostate. Normally, when the dissection is proceeding well you will not see the prerectal fatty tissue, which is covered by Denonvilliers' fascia. The blunt dissection is continued as far as possible towards the apex of the prostate, strictly in the midline, in order to avoid injury to the neurovascular bundles.

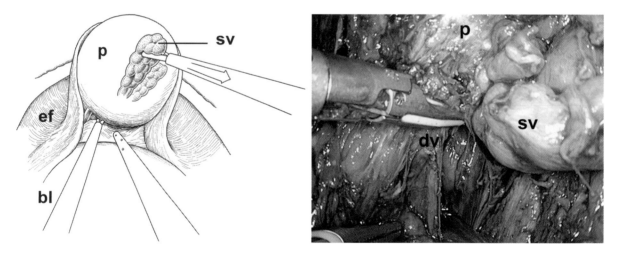

Complete mobilisation of Denonvilliers' fascia and all adhesive tissue is performed in the lateral direction to gain medial access to the prostatic pedicle and neurovascular bundles. The rectum is continuously pushed down by the assistant.

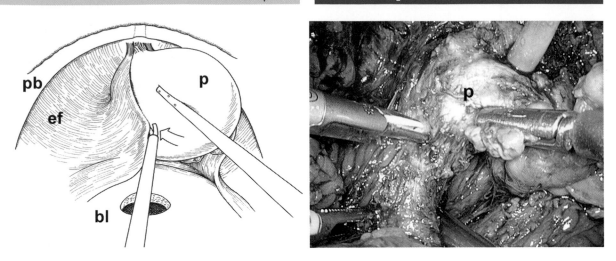

7

The mobilisation of the periprostatic fascia from the prostatic capsule is continued, by blunt and sharp dissection, in order to gain lateral access to the prostatic pedicles and the neurovascular bundles. For this step the prostate must be pushed laterally by the assistant.

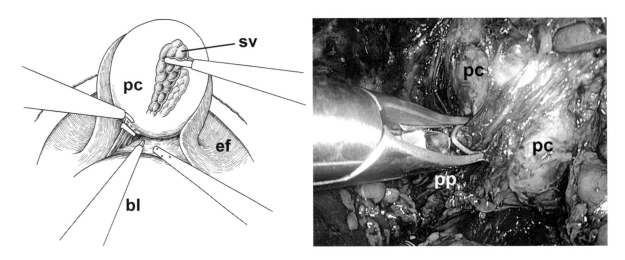

At this point of the procedure we have created two safe planes. Medially as well as laterally the "shining" surface of the prostatic capsule is clearly seen. If you lose orientation, always go back to these safe planes. The prostate is now free from its surrounding fascias and is anchored by the pedicles and the apex. Traction on the left seminal vesicle is made contralaterally by pulling out of the pelvis. The left prostatic pedicle is clearly seen, is clipped (10 mm Endoclip II ML, Tyco) and divided very close to the surface of the prostate.

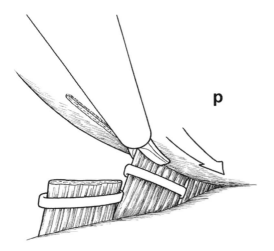
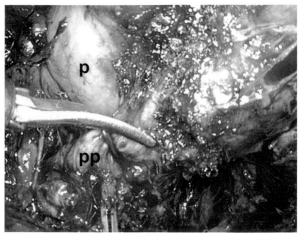

The prostatic pedicle must be clipped and cut step by step. It is not possible to include the entire pedicle within one clip. Care has to be taken to avoid inadvertent injury to the neurovascular bundle. It is advisable to advance the clipping and cutting in small steps. When the left-side dissection is completed, the same process is repeated on the right side. The surgeon uses the scissors with his right hand and the grasper with his left hand.

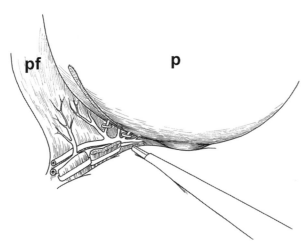
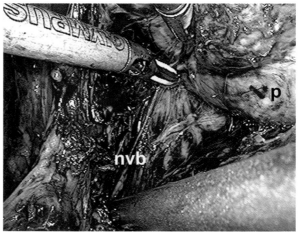

When the main prostatic pedicle has been fully dissected the remaining neurovascular bundle and periprostatic fascia can be detached from the prostatic capsule, in most cases bluntly. The assistant retracts the left seminal vesicle with his right-hand forceps and pushes the lateral side of the prostate with the instrument in his left hand. The prostate is thus slightly rotated. Small capsular vessels can be clipped with small clips (5 mm Endoclip, Tyco) and divided. The blunt dissection can be completed on both sides to free the entire posterior and posterolateral surface of the prostate. The SonoSurg device is only used for blunt dissection to avoid damage to the nerve structures. The posterior aspect of the apex can be seen when the blunt dissection is completed.

Especially in big prostates it can be difficult to gain access to the neurovascular bundles at the apex. It can be helpful for the surgeon to insert his right-hand instrument into one of the trocars of the right side, when access to the right neurovascular bundle is necessary. Alternatively, for this part of the procedure he may move to the right side of the patient and the assistant to the left.

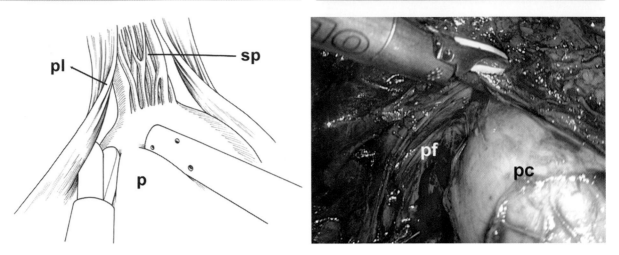

7

The prostate is now pushed into the pelvis contralaterally to provide good access to the apex and the urethra. The mobilised puboprostatic ligaments and the remaining puboprostatic fascia on the lateral surface of the prostate are now completely detached from the urethra and the apex. The assistant pulls the prostate to the right side for preparation of the left neurovascular bundle and vice versa. This dissection is performed bluntly. Only the ventral tissue upon the prostate is dissected with the SonoSurg. If bleeding occurs from branches of the Santorini plexus or from the Santorini plexus itself, coagulation should not be attempted (ligation of the plexus is the next step).

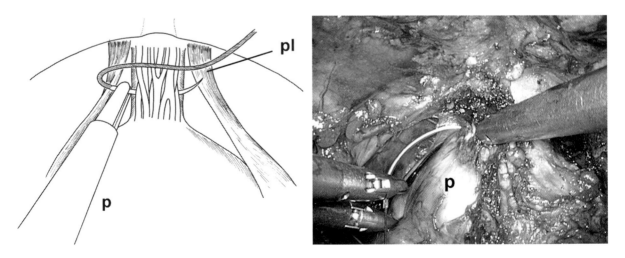

After full mobilisation the Santorini plexus is clearly visible from the lateral side. A 2–0 Polysorb GS-22 needle (slightly straightened) is then used and guided from left to right in the plane below the dorsal venous complex, and the plexus is thus ligated. During this step the assistant pushes the prostate dorsocranially to elongate the urethra.

7.5 Apical Dissection

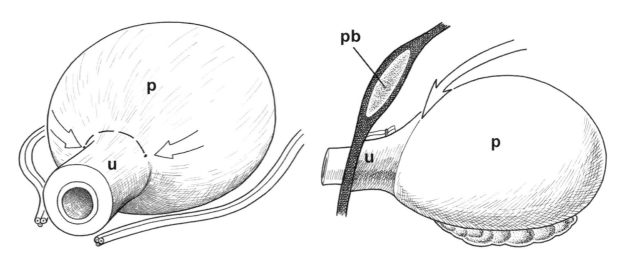

These two diagrams demonstrate the principles of apical dissection. It is always easier to find the border between apex and urethral laterally instead of ventrally (*left image*). The dissection is performed with Metzenbaum scissors, respecting the shape of the prostate and the course of the external sphincter, which overlaps the prostate ventrally, to protect as many striated muscle fibres of the external sphincter as possible. Note that the prostate extends more dorsally than ventrally. For this reason the dissection is not perpendicular. A strictly perpendicular dissection would leave residual prostatic tissue dorsally and could generate positive margins.

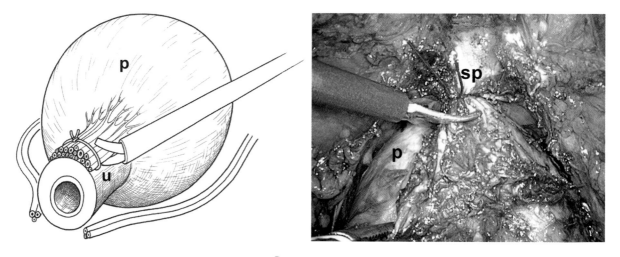

The apical dissection is a three-step procedure. It starts with the dissection of the Santorini plexus (step 1 of apical dissection). This is performed from lateral to medial, from left to right, until full dissection is completed. If the ligation of the venous complex is loosened or released during dissection of the complex, use a 2–0 Polysorb on a GU-46 needle to stitch and ligate the plexus again. The reason for the use of a GU-46 (5/8) needle is the retraction within the pelvic venous complex. One needs to suture deeper than previously to secure haemostasis.

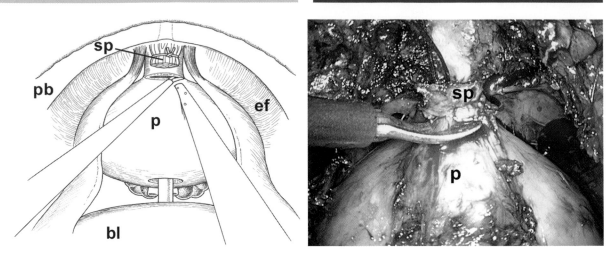

After the Santorini plexus is dissected the border between the prostate and the urethra (external sphincter) is found laterally at the 9 and 3 o'clock positions. The dissection converges medially from both sides (step 2 of apical dissection). For the entire apical dissection make sure that the catheter is inserted within the urethra and visible at the proximal prostatic end.

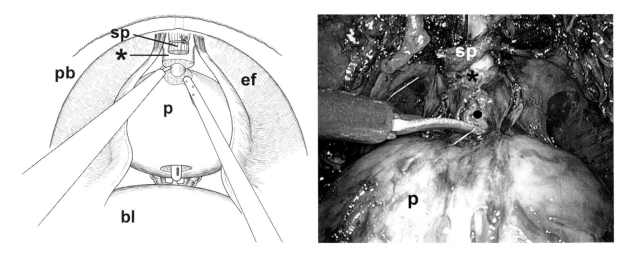

The urethra with the external sphincter (*star*) is dissected from the apex in small, carefully performed steps ventrally and laterally. For optimal access the prostate should once again be pushed dorsocranially by the assistant. Minor bleeding can be controlled with bipolar forceps if necessary. Extensive coagulation should be avoided. The smooth muscular inner layer of the urethra (*dot*) should be completely exposed ventrally and laterally. Cold scissors are exclusively used for all these steps.

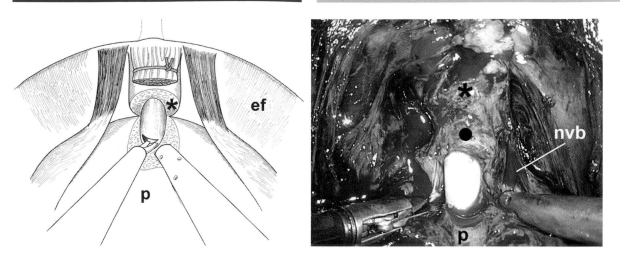

By pushing the prostate craniocaudally a longer segment of the smooth urethra (*dot*) is achieved. Dissection of the anterior urethra is then performed proximally very close to the prostate to preserve the urethra as long as possible (step 3 of apical dissection). The urethral catheter is now visible.

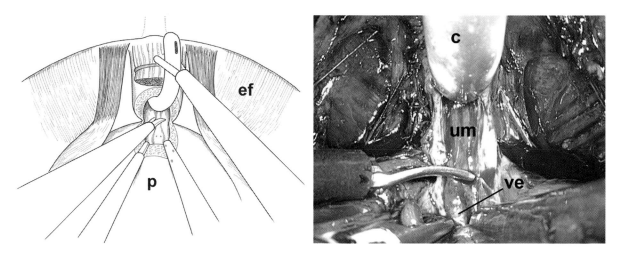

The assistant retracts the catheter towards the symphysis with the forceps on his right hand, and pushes the prostate down with the suction in his left hand. The urethral mucosa and the seminal colliculus (verumontanum) are now clearly visible. The dissection of the posterior urethra starts distally to the verumontanum.

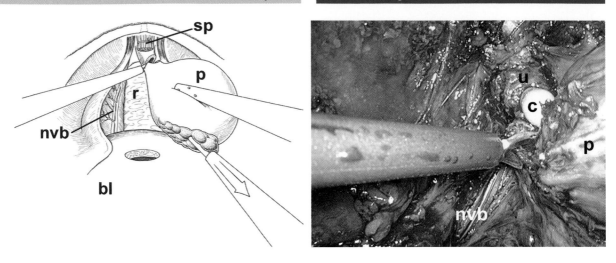

The final detachment of the posterior urethra is performed dorsolaterally to avoid any injury to the neurovascular bundles and the rectum. The assistant retracts the seminal vesicle contralaterally out of the pelvis and also pushes the prostate dorsolaterally.

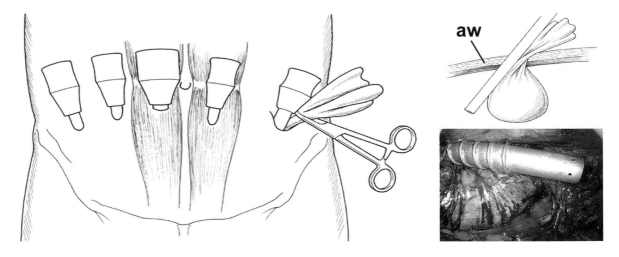

When the prostate is completely dissected from its adjacent structures, it is then placed in an endoscopic retrieval bag. The bag containing the prostatic specimen is partly extracted through the 12-mm trocar site and clamped. The trocar is then repositioned parallel to the bag, which is located in the left iliac fossa.

Alternatively, the endoscopic bag containing the specimen can be retracted through the 12-mm trocar site at this point of the procedure, especially if a positive margin is suspected. The skin and fascial incision is enlarged, depending on the size of the prostate. The suspicious margin on the specimen should be marked with colour and send for frozen section. After specimen extraction the fascia has to be sutured and the trocar repositioned to continue with the anastomosis.

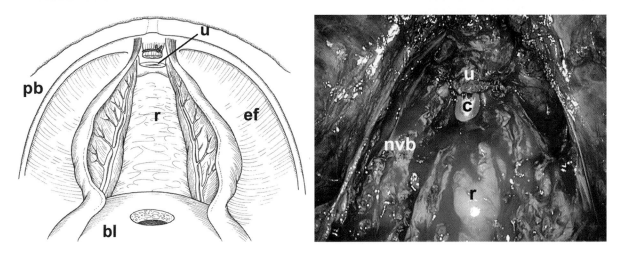

This picture shows the intraoperative field after complete detachment of the prostate in the case of bilateral nerve-sparing prostatectomy. The preserved neurovascular bundles are seen bilaterally. The intrafascial dissection technique offers a maximum of protection to the neurovascular bundles, leaving intact not only the neurovascular bundles but also the puboprostatic ligaments, the endopelvic fascia, and the periprostatic fascia (intrafascial dissection).

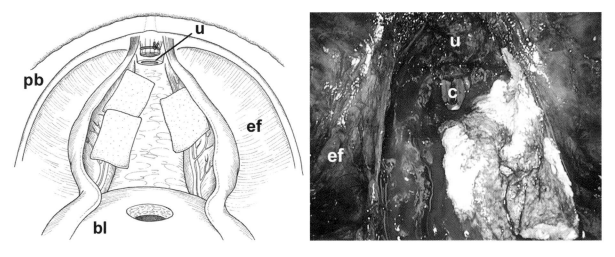

When there is minor bleeding from the neurovascular bundle (surface haemorrhage and slow venous oozing), use TachoSil® (Nycomed Austria GmbH). Technically it is easier to cut a large sponge (9.5×4.8 cm) of TachoSil® into two or three pieces than to use the whole sponge. Each piece of TachoSil® is carefully folded with the active yellow side on the outside and introduced through the 12-mm port. Alternatively, the sponge can be introduced with the help of a laparoscopic introducer sheath. When inside, then unfold and position it within the prostatic fossa overlaying the neurovascular bundles with the yellow active side in direct contact with the bleeding site. Pressure has to be applied for 3–5 min. Arterial bleeding cannot be prevented by any haemostatic; clips must be used in this case.

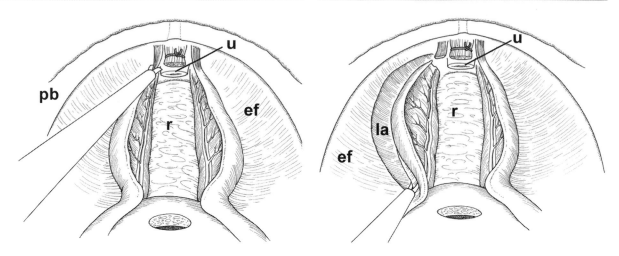

7

When the periprostatic fascia and the neurovascular bundle cannot be easily separated off the prostate, local tumour infiltration should be considered. An intraoperative frozen section of the area should be made. If the frozen section is positive, a wide excision procedure should be performed on the same side. The dissection starts with the puboprostatic ligament. Then, the endopelvic fascia should be widely excised from the apex to the level of the bladder neck.

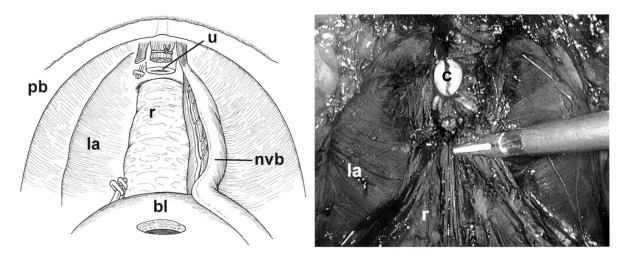

The tissue containing the fascias and the neurovascular bundle should be dissected both proximally and distally, with the aid of the SonoSurg device, mimicking the wide excision technique. Alternatively, you can use clipping and cold knife dissection. The same can be performed on the right side if necessary.

7.6 Anastomosis

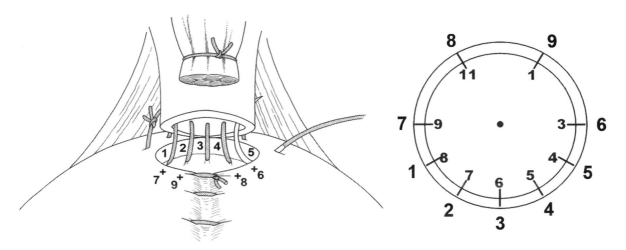

In principle the anastomosis can be performed with an interrupted or with a running suture. We prefer the interrupted suture technique. Depending on the size of the bladder neck, eight or nine sutures are necessary for a watertight anastomosis. In the case of a widely open bladder neck, bladder neck closure (ventrally) should also be performed. The sequence of stitches is clearly shown in the *left image*. In the *right image* the clock position of each stitch is marked (*internal numbers*). The *external numbers* show the suturing sequence.

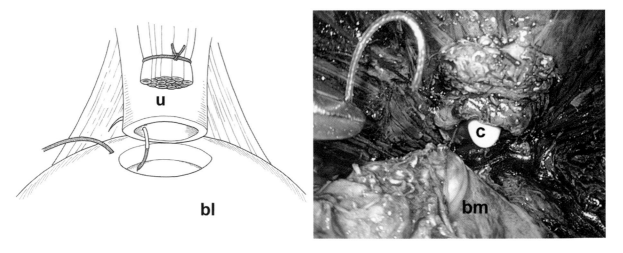

The anastomosis is performed with a 2–0 Polysorb suture on a GU-46 needle (alternative: UR-6 needle, 2–0 Vicryl). The bladder neck is always stitched first. All stitches are performed "outside-in" at the bladder neck and "inside-out" at the urethra. In this way the sutures are always tied extraluminally. The first stitch starts at the 8 o'clock position (backhand–backhand). When starting the anastomosis the Trendelenburg position is reduced to a minimum required.

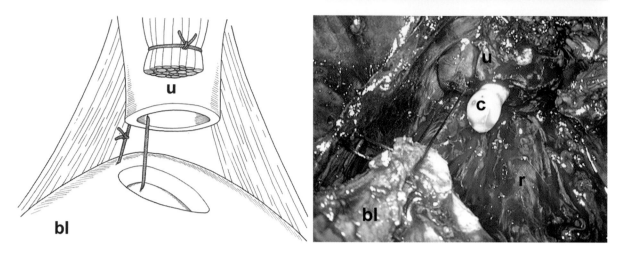

7

In the very rare case of tension on the urethra, try first to change the patient's position by bringing his head up. If this does not help, do not attempt to approximate the bladder to the urethra in one step. Secure the knot of the first suture before full approximation. Make sure that the bladder is empty. The final approximation can be reached with the next stitch.

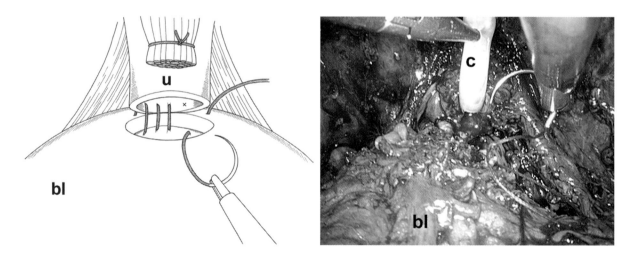

The next stitches are positioned at the 7, 6 and 5 o'clock positions (forehand at the bladder neck, backhand at the urethra). When stitching the urethra during the posterior anastomosis the urethral catheter always needs to be lifted up by the assistant or the surgeon to guide suture positioning. After each urethral stitch, the catheter needs to be pulled back in order to rule out inadvertent fixation by the anastomotic suture.

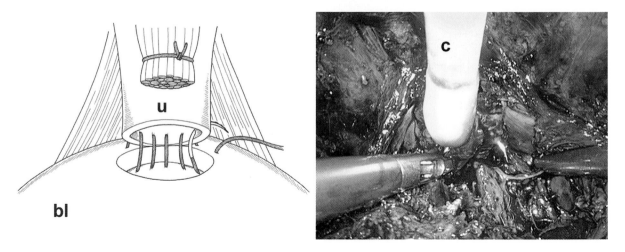

The 4 o'clock stitch is then done forehand (bladder neck)–forehand (urethra). In nerve-sparing procedures take care not to include in the suturing the neurovascular bundles (especially the 8 and 4 o'clock stitches are dangerous). The assistant should guide the stitch with the help of the suction, as shown in the endoscopic image.

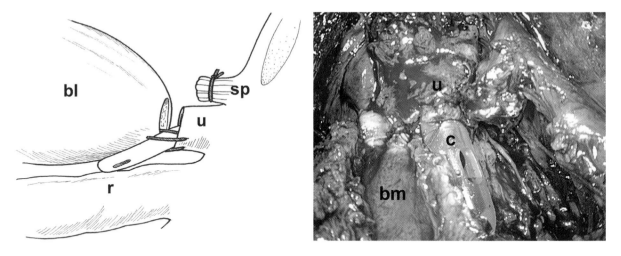

After the dorsal circumference has been completed, the final silicone catheter (18–20 F) is placed into the bladder. This is the test for the quality of the posterior part of the anastomosis. If there is a problem the catheter does not slide into the bladder and finds its way through the stitches behind the bladder, as shown in the diagram. You then have to revise the anastomosis.

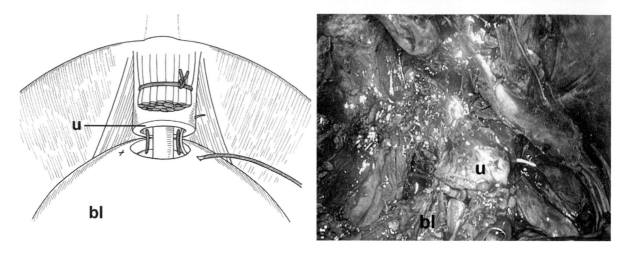

7

The anastomosis is now continued laterally on both sides. On the left side (9 o'clock) the stitches are thrown backhand–backhand and on the right side (3 o'clock) forehand–forehand, as shown. These stitches are relatively easy to perform and should be performed in one step (stitch the bladder and urethra in one move).

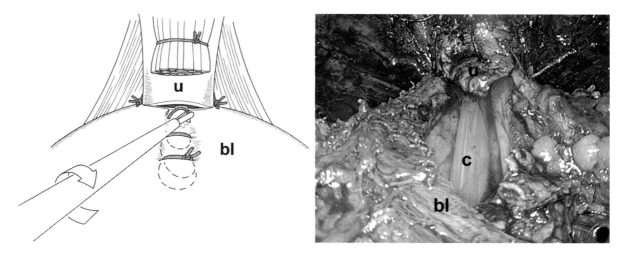

If during the bladder neck dissection a bladder neck-preserving technique is not feasible, a bladder neck reconstruction at a 12 o'clock position is deemed necessary at this point. Use a running suture with the same needle and suture material. Alternatively, single stitches can be placed. Make sure that the stitches are full thickness on the bladder wall.

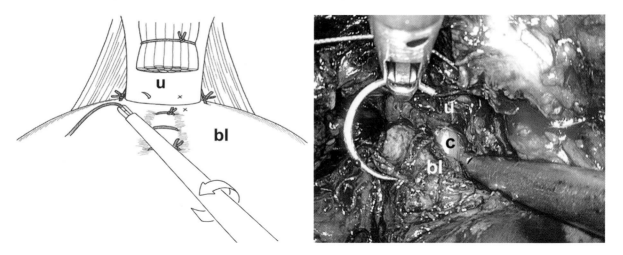

The final two anastomotic sutures are placed at 11 and 1 o'clock positions (left side: backhand–backhand, right side: forehand–forehand). For the 11 o'clock stitch the needle holder is introduced through the right medial 5-mm trocar (on the assistant's side). This stitch is thrown backhand at the bladder neck and backhand at the urethra, and can be performed in one or two moves. For knot tying the needle holder is moved back to its initial position.

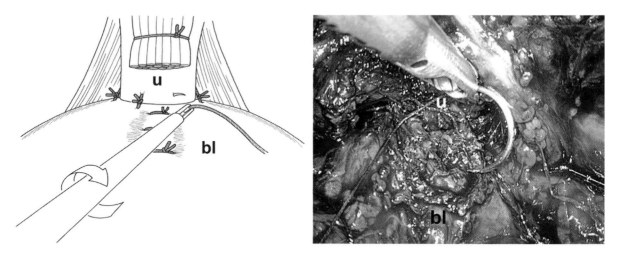

When suturing the urethra these stitches (11 o'clock and 1 o'clock) should not include the whole tissue of the urethra. They should embrace the Santorini plexus, connective tissue and puboprostatic ligament (not through the mucosa and the musculature of the urethra), thus avoiding any damage to the external (urethral) sphincter and its blood supply and finally fixing the "new" bladder neck to its anatomical position (not shown).

    After conclusion of the stitching process the catheter must be moved to make sure that there is no entrapment within the suture lines (very rare). The water-tightness of the anastomosis is finally checked by filling the bladder with 200 ml sterile water. Lateral and ventral leaks can be managed by additional suturing. In the case of a major posterior leak the anastomosis needs to be opened and performed again.

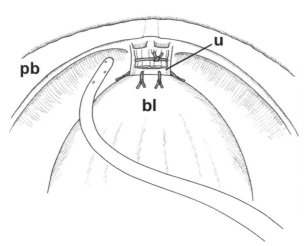

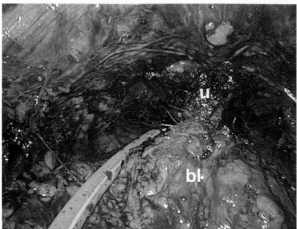

At the end of the procedure, a 16-F Robinson drainage catheter is placed into the retropubic space on the left side of the anastomosis. We do not recommend the placement of the drainage on top of the anastomosis. Finally, the endoscopic bag containing the specimen is retracted through the 12-mm trocar site at the end of the procedure. Depending on the size of the prostate the skin and fascia incision may have to be enlarged. The drain is removed 24–48 h after the procedure. Five days postoperatively cystography is performed, and if there is no anastomotic leak the urethral catheter is removed.

7.7 EERPE and Hernia Repair with Mesh Placement

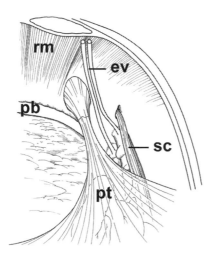

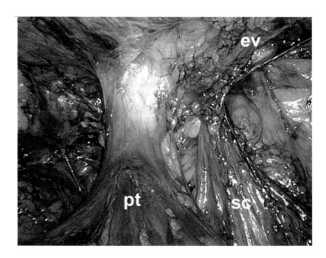

In approximately 5–8% of patients treated with EERPE there is a need for concomitant repair of unilateral or bilateral inguinal hernia. We prefer a standardised totally extraperitoneal technique, which uses the principle of tensionless hernia repair, overlaying the entire myopectineal orifice with one large piece of mesh. A 10×15-cm polypropylene mesh is placed in the preperitoneal space covering both direct and indirect hernial orifices at the end of the prostatectomy. The technique is described here.

In direct hernias, the hernial sac (peritoneum) is found medial to the epigastric vessels.

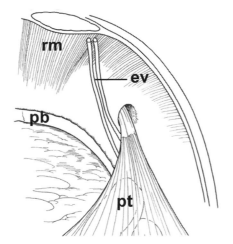 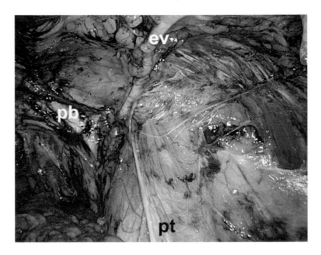

In indirect hernias, the peritoneal sac travels on the anteromedial aspect of the spermatic cord as it enters the internal ring. The hernial sac should be carefully retracted and dissected free from the cord. Care is taken to avoid injury of the hernial sac (peritoneum), its containing structures and the vessels of the spermatic cord.

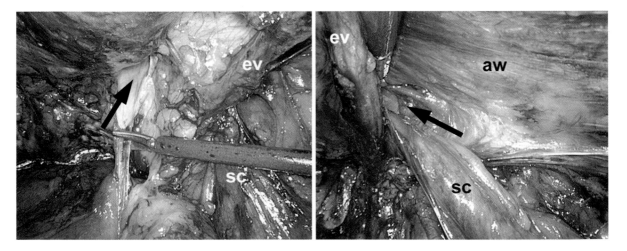

Traction and counter-traction are used to reduce the hernial sac. Especially the medial fascial defect becomes clearly visible after dissection (*arrow, left image*). In some patients the dissection of the medial hernial sac is nearly completely accomplished by the balloon during initial dissection of the preperitoneal space. In indirect hernias, after dissection of the hernial sac the inguinal ring (*arrow, right image*) is clearly seen. In all hernias, the hernial sac must be dissected before starting the prostatectomy and the actual hernia repair is performed after the completion of the anastomosis.

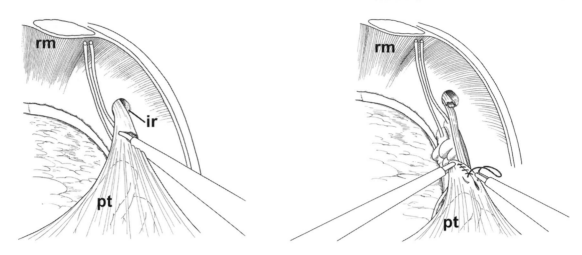

7

If the hernia sac cannot be completely and sufficiently retracted (i.e. large indirect inguinal–scrotal hernia), the hernial sac can be divided at the level of the internal inguinal ring. Care should be taken during the incision not to injure the bowel within the hernial sac. Closure of any peritoneal defect is essential at the site of the hernia repair. Contact between bowel and the mesh would cause adhesions and probably ileus. For this reason minor and larger defects should be closed by suturing.

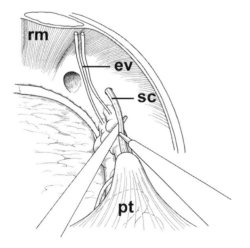

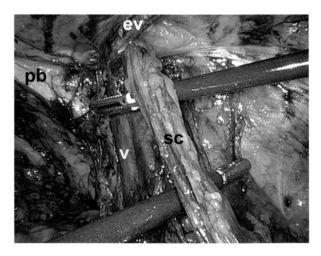

The entire spermatic cord is elevated and an opening is created posteriorly for the insertion of the mesh. Most of the dissection is performed bluntly. This space should not be too small to avoid folding of the mesh once in place.

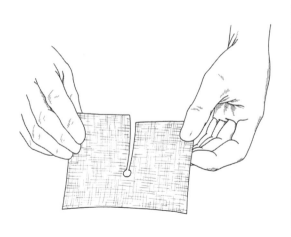
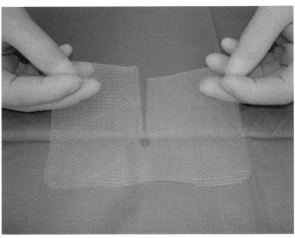

Extracorporeal preparation of the Prolene mesh (9–10×14–15 cm) is performed. A 6-cm incision is made in the middle of the mesh, and a 0.5-cm hole is cut out for the spermatic cord. When a large medial hernia is being repaired, the medial aspect of the mesh should be larger.

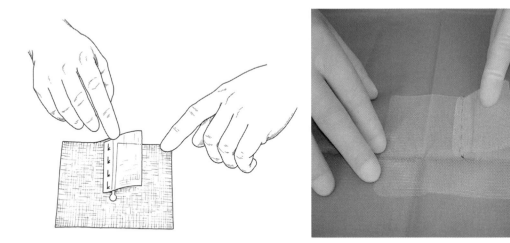

The incision in the mesh is covered by a further 4×6-cm Prolene mesh. This additional patch is secured with a 2–0 Prolene running suture. The suture should not be under tension to avoid shrinkage of the mesh.

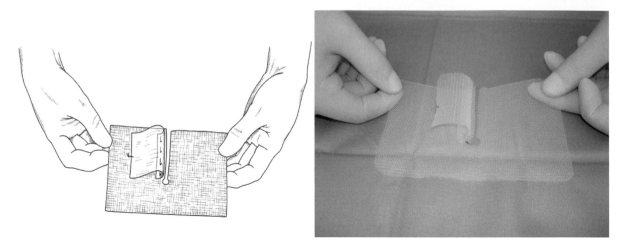

7

In the next steps, the mesh is inserted and placed around the spermatic cord. The flap is temporarily fixed at the medial aspect of the main mesh by a stay suture. This suture should be loose to facilitate later intracorporeal cutting.

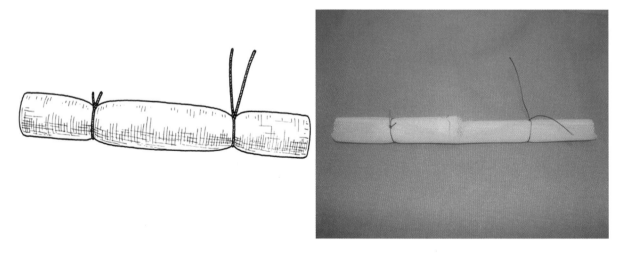

The mesh is rolled up and fixed by two stay sutures. A long suture is used for the *l*ateral aspect (*l*=*l*ong) and a short suture for the medial aspect of the mesh. This enables easy recognition and placement in situ.

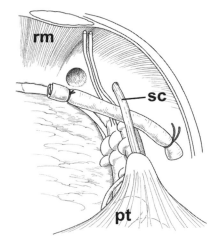
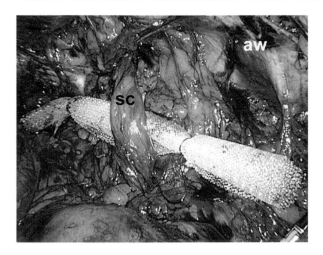

This preparation of the mesh roll was necessary to facilitate mesh placement through the 12-mm trocar in the preperitoneal space. The introduced mesh is placed under the spermatic cord. Note that the side with the long suture should be placed laterally.

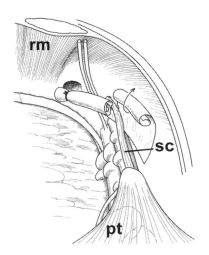
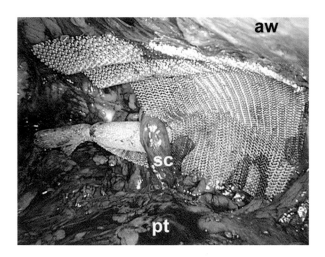

The stay sutures are cut in sequence. The lateral (long) stay suture is cut first and the lateral part of the mesh is completely unfolded. Make sure that the lateral part of the mesh is completely unfolded and there is no shrinkage or kinking.

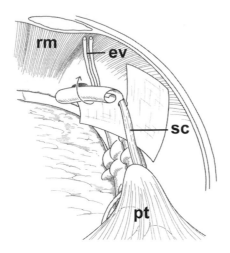

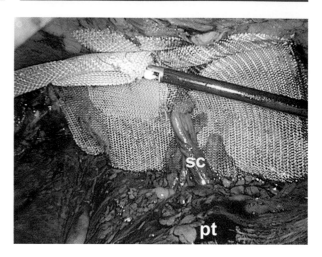

7

The medial (short) stay suture is then cut and the medial part of the mesh is unfolded. This medial part slightly overlaps the lateral part of the mesh. The assistant should now hold the mesh in place with his instrument.

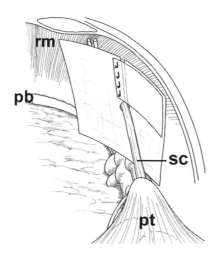

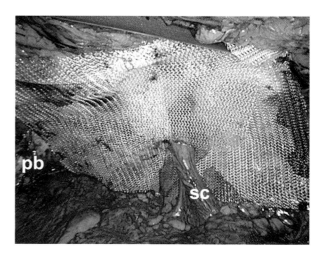

The stay suture of the flap is now cut and the flap is unfolded overlapping the lateral part of the mesh. Thus, the mesh is positioned around the spermatic cord to cover the hernial orifices and the entire space from the symphysis pubis in the midline to the anterior superior iliac spine laterally. In the case of bilateral hernias, two pieces of mesh are used and overlapped. After release of the carbon dioxide from the preperitoneal space at the end of the procedure, the mesh is anchored to the abdominal wall by intra-abdominal pressure alone. Placing the mesh around the spermatic cord prevents any possibility of its dislocating or migrating. Staples or stitches are not used for fixation of the mesh.

Troubelshooting

8

Jens-Uwe Stolzenburg · Minh Do · Robert Rabenalt · Anja Dietel · Heidemarie Pfeiffer ·
Frank Reinhardt · Michael C. Truss · Evangelos Liatsikos

Contents

Endoscopic extraperitoneal radical prostatectomy (EERPE) has been developed profoundly, and standardised to a point that it has become the first-line option for patients with localised prostate cancer in an increasing number of institutions. The incidence of most complications correlates directly with the surgeon's experience, and the various complications are related to technical errors rather than to the technique itself.

Increasing experience significantly reduces the occurrence of complications. Furthermore, minimising laparoscopic complications requires a skilled operating team. A well-trained assistant and camera operator are of paramount importance. Disorientation and unclear anatomy are the origins of most complications in minimally invasive surgery.

This chapter focuses on the identification, management and prevention of the most common complications associated with EERPE. The laparoscopist, as well as the robotic surgeon, should be able to recognise promptly, treat efficiently, and ideally prevent most complications of EERPE.

8.1 Intraoperative Problems

8.1.1 Creation of Preperitoneal Space and Trocar Placement

8.1.1.1 Balloon Trocar Placed Intraperitoneally

The balloon dissection is always performed under direct visual control. One will realise very quickly if the balloon trocar is within the peritoneal cavity. In that case extract the trocar, ignore the hole in the peritoneal cavity, and try once again to dissect carefully with your finger parallel to the posterior rectus fascia to gain access to the extraperitoneal space. It might be helpful to enlarge the skin incision to permit easier and safer access to the anatomical landmarks (posterior rectus sheath).

8.1.1.2 Rupture of Balloon Itself

When there is a rupture of the balloon itself (very rare), remember to remove all its segments. This should be done after the full development of the extraperitoneal space. Furthermore, all trocars should

be placed, especially the 10-mm trocar in the left iliac fossa. This trocar is large enough to remove sizable remnant pieces of the balloon trocar. It makes no sense to try to remove the balloon pieces through a 5-mm trocar.

8.1.1.3 Rupture of Peritoneum During Dissection of Extraperitoneal Space

When during the dissection of the extraperitoneal space there is inadvertent opening into the peritoneal cavity, there is no need for panic. This can happen particularly if the patient has had previous pelvic surgery (e.g. appendectomy, hernia repair). Continue the dissection and proceed with the operation. If the extraperitoneal space is significantly reduced, consult the anaesthetist for muscle relaxation. In most cases of reduced extraperitoneal space, insufficient muscle relaxation is the cause of the event. If the problem persists, consider opening a wider „window" (very seldom necessary) to the peritoneum and there should be no further problems. If the dissection of the peritoneum cannot be completely performed due to extensive adhesions, one should incise the peritoneum and create a „window" deliberately, allowing for safe trocar insertion (also very seldom necessary).

8.1.1.4 Tips for Safe Trocar Placement

All trocars should be placed under direct visual control. Additionally, the Hassan trocar must not be advanced all the way in the working space and should be partially retracted during trocar placement.

In difficult cases (i.e. obese patients, extensive adhesions) the use of a fine needle to prepuncture and visualise the site of planned trocar insertion into the preperitoneum is sometimes useful. Assistance with the suction tube, from a pre-existing port, exerting pressure toward the inner surface of the abdominal wall at the point of desired trocar insertion, also helps to avoid damage to vascular structures. The trocar is then forwarded without its internal trocar sliding over the suction tube within the extraperitoneal space.

Special trocars have been designed mounted on a prepuncturing needle to facilitate trocar insertion (Versastep, Tyco). The needle is covered with a special mesh. When the final position has been reached, the needle is extracted and an internal 5- or 10-mm blunt-tip trocar is inserted through the mesh into the extraperitoneal space. The trocar dilates the tract within the mesh and eventually reaches its final diameter.

8.1.1.5　Bowel Injury During Trocar Placement

Bowel injury is one of the most severe complications of EERPE because it is potentially life threatening, especially if not recognised intraoperatively.

Unrecognised perforation usually presents within 24–72 h after surgery, and thermal injury often presents 6–10 days postoperatively. The presenting symptoms may be non-specific, including vomiting, abdominal pain, distension, presence of bubbles within the urine, faecaluria and/or malaise. Fever and leucocytosis are present and septic shock may develop. Thus, any patient presenting with persistent abdominal pain, nausea, or general malaise within 2 weeks of EERPE should be evaluated carefully to exclude bowel injury. Patients and general practitioners should also be advised to promptly report symptoms, avoiding potential detrimental effects of misdiagnosed bowel injury.

Laceration of the bowel can be caused by the insertion of the lateral trocars if peritoneal adhesions to the lateral wall have not been adequately mobilised. In the case of trocar-associated laceration, the injury may escape detection. Meticulous and thorough mobilisation of the lateral attachments of the peritoneum to the retroperitoneal space must be performed before positioning of the lateral trocars. No mention of bowel injury due to trocar insertion is found in the literature associated with EERPE. It is more a theoretical risk, but nevertheless the surgeon needs to be aware of this potential complication. In cases in which the peritoneum cannot be safely reflected, incision of the peritoneum for better visualisation of the trocars is suggested.

8.1.1.6　Injury of Bladder During Dissection of Extraperitoneal Space

Inadvertent bladder injury can occur during dissection of the extraperitoneal space, especially in patients with a prior history of extraperitoneal hernioplasty with mesh placement. When identified, it should be repaired in a single layer. Leakage should be ruled out by infusing 200 ml saline into the bladder. We have encountered two intraoperative bladder injuries, both in patients with previous hernioplasty mesh insertion.

8.1.2　Bleeding

8.1.2.1　Bleeding from Epigastric Vessels

Injury of the inferior epigastric vessels is the most common vascular complication and is often recognised intraoperatively.

Injury to the epigastric vessels is usually caused during insertion of the fourth trocar (pararectal line, right iliac fossa) and can be avoided by careful inspection of the abdominal wall via the laparoscope before trocar insertion (see Chap. 7). Furthermore, the use of a fine needle to prepuncture and visualise the site of planned trocar insertion into the preperitoneum is sometimes useful (Versaport, Tyco). If the vessels are damaged, bipolar coagulation and clipping are often effective means to control bleeding. When bleeding is persistent, suturing with the aid of a straight needle through the abdominal wall, encaging the bleeding vessel, is very useful (Fig. 8.1). The suture is released 2 days after the initial operative procedure. Nevertheless, gas insufflation pressure may tamponade bleeding intraoperatively, and this may not become apparent until after trocar removal. Meticulous inspection of all trocar sites for active bleeding before final laparoscope removal, after the extraperitoneal CO_2 pressure has been lowered, is strongly recommended. In addition, the laparoscope should be inserted through the 12-mm left lateral trocar, facilitating direct inspection of the right trocar extraction and any possible injury to the epigastric vessels.

8.1.2.2　Venous Bleeding

When venous bleeding occurs one should always increase the pressure to 20 mmHg, clean the operative field with the suction and control the bleeding with the use of the bipolar forceps.

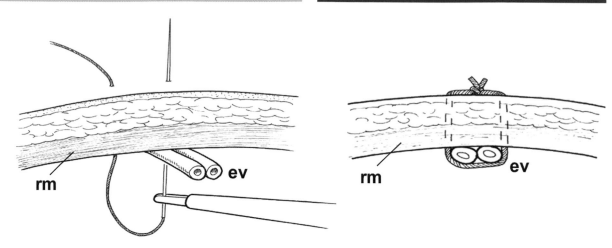

Fig. 8.1. Suturing of persistently bleeding epigastric vessels. A straight long needle is inserted outside-in from the skin to the extraperitoneal space. The needle is then grasped with forceps and needle holder and advanced inside-out to the skin, entrap-ping the bleeding vessels. The knot is positioned extracorpore-ally. This manoeuvre can be repeated. Two days after the EERPE the suture can be released

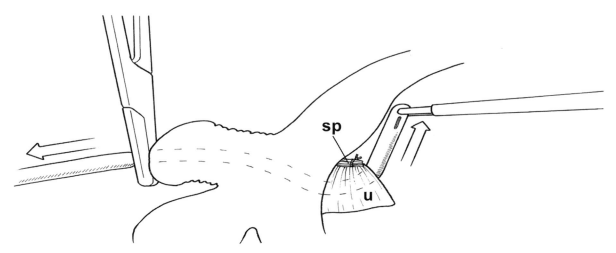

Fig. 8.2. Management of persistent bleeding from the Santorini plexus. After complete apical dissection (or after complete dissection of the ventral circumference of the junction between the urethra and the apex of the prostate) the assistant grasps the urethral catheter and exerts traction ventrally (towards the symphysis). Traction has to be applied on the catheter for 5–10 min, from the outside manually or with the help of a clamp

8.1.2.3 Arterial Bleeding

Arterial bleeding cannot be controlled by increasing the gas pressure. By good teamwork, sources of bleeding have to be identified and controlled by clipping and suturing, or by coagulation. The surgeon should first grasp the bleeding vessel to stop bleeding, then clean the field with the suction, and finally bring the haemorrhage under control.

8.1.2.4 Santorini Plexus

Haemorrhage may also arise from Santorini's venous plexus, which can be avoided by adequate ligation of the plexus (see Chap. 7), although it may still occur during apical dissection. An initial increase of gas insufflation to a pressure of 20 mmHg is suggested. Subsequently, meticulous bipolar coagulation should be performed without any damage to the sphincteric fibres and neurovascular bundles (NVBs). We recommend additional suturing instead of extensive use of bipolar coagulation. We prefer to use a 2–0 Polysorb suture on a GU-46 needle for better manoeuvrability.

In the case of persistent bleeding, the ventral urethral wall is completely dissected and the catheter is retracted with tension by the assistant for approximately 5–10 min to tamponade bleeding (Fig. 8.2). During the waiting period one has sufficient time to inspect the operative field and plan for eventual further suturing if needed. At the end of the procedure, reduction of insufflation pressure is recommended to allow identification of bleeding vessels.

8.1.2.5 Injury of Iliac Vein

The external iliac vein is also at risk of injury during EERPE. Damage may be caused either during lymph node dissection, or by vigorous insertion of instruments without visual control. If this injury is identified intraoperatively, an experienced surgeon may be able to repair it endoscopically (4–0 Prolene), whilst a less experienced surgeon is advised to convert to an open procedure. In the latter case the CO_2 insufflation should be maintained or increased during conversion in order to minimise blood loss. It is noteworthy that increasing the gas insufflation pressure may effectively control venous bleeding, thus facilitating endoscopic repair. Make sure that when suturing the "collapsed" vein caused by the increased gas pressure, you do not suture the two sides of the vein together.

8.1.2.6 Bleeding from Neurovascular Bundles

A possible source of postoperative haematoma is small vessels adjacent to the NVBs. Intraoperative coagulation should be avoided. Management of bleeding close to the NVB area should be performed either by selective suturing or by using matrix haemostatic sealants. Some authors advocate the use of TachoSil (Nycomed, Austria) (see also Chap. 7) or FloSeal (Baxter Inc., Irvine, CA, USA) along the entire length of the NVB. It can be helpful to insert TachoSil and cover it with a dry sheet of haemostatic matrix (e.g. Gelfoam, Surgicel or Tabotamp) acting as a protective cover to keep it in place.

8.1.3 Ureteral Damage

8.1.3.1 Damage During Lymph Node Dissection

When extensive lymph node dissection is performed the ureter might be damaged, and/or partially or totally transected. If there is doubt that the ureter has been transected or damaged intraoperatively, indigo carmine and furosemide may be injected intravenously to check for leakage of dye through the ureter. We have never experienced a ureteral injury during extraperitoneal lymphadenectomy. This risk is more prominent during the laparoscopic transperitoneal approach, due to the close proximity of the working space to the ureters. The ureter can be mistaken for the vas.

8.1.3.2 Damage During Dissection of Posterior Bladder Neck

Ureteral damage can also be caused during the dissection of the posterior bladder neck and subsequent anastomosis. In the case of doubt regarding entrapment of the ureteral orifices during the anastomotic process, indigo carmine is administered to facilitate orifice visualisation. Intraoperative ureteral catheterisation is advised if the orifices are close to the anastomotic site, especially during the surgeon's learning curve.

In the case of prior transurethral resection of the prostate, the preoperative insertion of double pigtail stents is recommended, because the distance between the bladder neck and the ureteral orifices may be too short for safe dissection and anastomosis. In addition, the border between the prostatic cavity and the bladder neck may be difficult to identify.

In our series, we observed one case of intraoperative injury of the interureteric crest. A hydrophilic guidewire (Terumo) was inserted through the urethra and then endoscopically guided into the ureteral orifices (Fig. 8.3). Double pigtail stents were then inserted over the wire bilaterally to ascertain ureteral viability. In the case of doubt the use of fluoroscopy is suggested. The bladder neck was then reconstructed endoscopically at the 6 o'clock position.

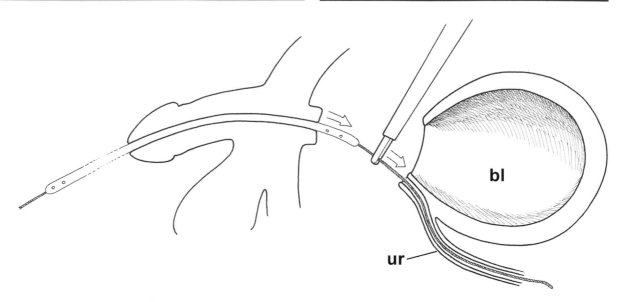

Fig. 8.3. Technique of intraoperative ureteral stenting. A 0.038′ hydrophilic guidewire (Terumo) is inserted through the urethra and guided with the help of two laparoscopic graspers into the ureteral orifice. Once the guidewire is in place, the double pigtail catheter is advanced over it within the ureter. This manoeuvre can be performed on both sides

8.1.3.3 Ureteral Obstruction

In our series of 1,500 EERPEs two patients presented postoperatively with anuria and were treated either by bilateral double pigtail catheterisation (n=1), or by bilateral percutaneous nephrostomy insertion (n=1). In both cases no cause of obstruction was identified during stenting or imaging of the ureters. The reason for the obstruction remains unclear, though we favour the idea of anastomotic oedema. When the ureteral orifice is very close to the anastomosis the oedema may cause temporary ureteral obstruction. Similar problems with postoperative anuria have been reported by others.

8.1.4 Problems with Bladder Neck Dissection

8.1.4.1 Intraprostatic Dissection

Before starting the posterior bladder neck dissection, make sure that the natural groove between bladder mucosa and prostate in the dorsal direction can be identified. It is of utmost importance that the assistant exerts traction on the catheter so the posterior bladder neck is ideally exposed.

In the case of intraprostatic dissection, stop the dissection, go back to the bladder, open the bladder ventrally and identify the ureteral orifices as landmarks of the bladder trigone. Then continue the dissection caudally to the orifices towards the rectum to find the right plane. Tangential dissection should be avoided. Alternatively, the correct plane can be found laterally by dissecting and cutting all lateral connections of the bladder and the prostate. It is always easier to dissect the posterior bladder neck when you expand the dissection laterally, freeing the prostate from the bladder. Note that the dissection needs to follow a perpendicular plane to ascertain access to the seminal vesicles. It is important to avoid oblique dissection because you will end up dissecting within the prostate.

8.1.4.2 Conversion

The main reason for conversion to open surgery (especially during the initial phase of the learning curve) is the loss of orientation when performing the posterior bladder neck dissection. Intraprostatic dissection may hinder the favourable oncologic outcome of the procedure, and thus one should remember that conversion need not be a source of shame; on the contrary, it can be a sign of wisdom.

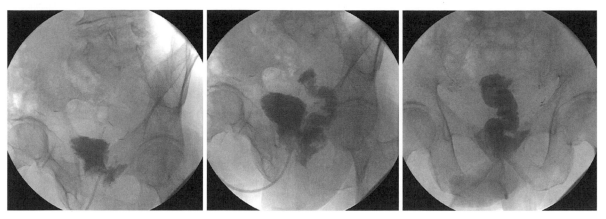

Fig. 8.4. Retrograde cystogram obtained on the 10th postoperative day, showing a rectourethral fistula. The initial cystography performed on the 5th postoperative day showed no sign of urine extravasation or fistula presence. The patient presented on the 10th day after the operation with air bubbles in his urine

8.1.5 Rectal Injury

Rectal injury can either occur during dissection (immediate injury) or be caused by extensive coagulation during the apical dissection. The majority of rectal injuries occur towards the end of the procedure when dissecting the apex dorsally, especially in patients with a previous history of prostatitis, fibrotic prostate, etc. Some authors advocate the use of intrarectal devices for better visualisation of the anterior rectal layer. In the case of doubts during dissection, the use of rectal insufflation with air in combination with filling of the operative field with water is recommended. Rectal injury will result in air bubbles, which can be easily detected. Prevention of such an untoward situation is achieved by meticulous dissection. If rectal injury is identified, endoscopic correction with a two-layer suture line must be performed. Afterwards, parenteral nutrition for at least 6 days is recommended. When a direct rectal injury is not recognised intraoperatively, patients tend to present with general signs of peritonitis and eventually sepsis during the first 3 days after surgery, and open surgical correction is necessary.

The incidence of rectal injury has been reported at between 0.5% and 9%. In our series, six patients sustained intraoperative rectal injuries, which were repaired endoscopically with a two-layer suture. One of these patients developed a rectourethral fistula (Fig. 8.4) requiring colostomy and secondary perineal repair.

8.1.6 Anastomotic Leaks

Intraoperative testing of the anastomosis to ensure no leakage is crucial. Seven to nine anastomotic sutures are required to perform a perfectly watertight anastomosis when performing interrupted sutures. Great care is taken to achieve a perfect posterior anastomotic layer, in order to avoid dorsal leakage. After completion of the anastomosis, the watertightness of the anastomosis is checked. Initially 100 ml of fluid are instilled into the bladder through the indwelling catheter. If a leak is found, depending on its origin we either perform additional anastomotic sutures (anterolateral leakage), or decide to redo the anastomosis (dorsal major leakage). If the leak cannot be managed by performing additional sutures, the anastomosis should be revised. If no leakage occurs, an additional 100 ml fluid should be injected via the transurethral catheter. In the case of minor leakage, tension can be applied on the catheter for 24 h to facilitate the healing process.

8.1.7 Gas Embolism

Gas embolism is a very rare but potentially life-threatening complication. Carbon dioxide may enter the venous vascular system and thereafter be trapped in the right ventricle, causing outflow obstruction from the right ventricle into the pulmonary artery. The initial clinical sign is a drop in end-tidal carbon dioxide concentration, as a result of decreased blood flow in the lungs. In case of suspected gas embolism, insufflation should be stopped immediately and cardiopulmonary resuscitation is required. Rolling the patient onto his left side facilitates expulsion of gas from the ventricle. During the past 6 years we have performed more than 2,000 laparoscopic procedures and have never experienced gas embolism.

8.2 Postoperative Problems

8.2.1 Bleeding/Haematoma

One of the advantages of the extraperitoneal access is that minor postoperative bleeding can stop by a natural tamponade effect. The postoperative detection of haematomas should be performed with the aid of ultrasonography. Very seldom is CT necessary.

If there is minor bleeding from the urethral catheter the balloon should be inflated with 20 ml and minor traction on the catheter should be applied. Nevertheless, if there is a postoperative bleeding that requires reintervention, the latter should be started endoscopically. The same port sites should be used. It is important to use a 10-mm suction tube (see Chap. 3.1) to be able to aspirate all the clots from the operative field. After aspiration the site of haemorrhage is identified and dealt with. In our experience, the majority of these cases could be handled endoscopically. At the end of the procedure reduce the gas pressure gradually (12 mmHg – 10 mmHg – 8 mmHg - 6 mmHg) and wait 1–2 min between the steps to de-

tect bleeding previously tamponaded by the gas pressure. If bleeding cannot be controlled, do not hesitate to convert to an open surgical procedure.

8.2.2 Catheter Blockage

Urine drainage can be impaired postoperatively by blood clot formation, which may potentially jeopardise the anastomosis. If postoperative haematuria is present, it is useful to force diuresis to prevent clotting. Lavage of the catheter and bladder with slow irrigation is recommended. Traction on the catheter may also be helpful. In addition, ward staff should be aware of this potential complication to ensure early detection.

During our initial experience with laparoscopic transperitoneal prostatectomy, we had one patient with persisting gross haematuria. Endoscopic transurethral inspection on day 2 revealed bleeding vessels at the bladder neck that were coagulated successfully. In such rare cases cystoscopy and electrofulguration of the bleeding vessel is advised.

Figure 8.5 shows a cystogram on the 5th postoperative day with no anastomotic leak but with a big intravesical blood clot. The patient presented slight haematuria immediately after the operation, but the urine cleared during the 2nd day after operation. The clot was adherent to the anastomosis and could not be removed through the urethral catheter. Immediately after cystography and catheter removal, cystoscopy was performed for clot removal. The follow-up was uneventful.

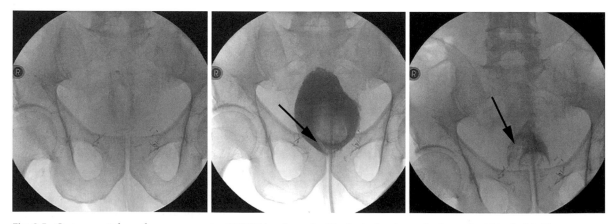

Fig. 8.5. Cystogram 5 days after nerve-sparing EERPE (performed with clips), showing a clot (arrow) within the bladder

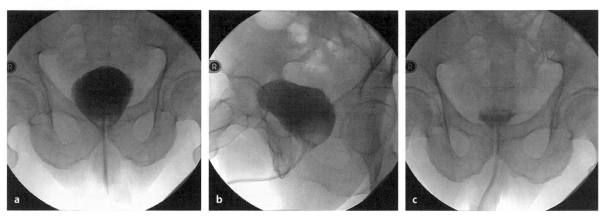

Fig. 8.6. Normal cystogram with 100 ml contrast media 5 days postoperatively. Cystography should comprise a minimum of four steps: (1) X-ray without contrast media (not shown); (2) X-ray with anterior-posterior projection (**a**); (3) X-ray with lateral projection (**b**); (4) X-ray with emptied bladder (**c**)

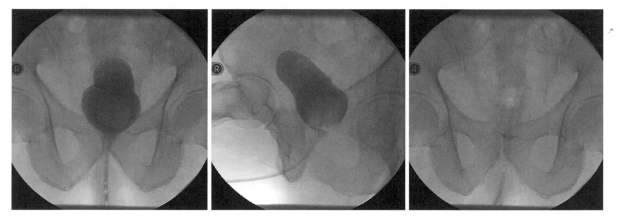

Fig. 8.7. Normal cystogram 5 days postoperatively in a patient with a widely open bladder neck during prostatectomy, requiring bladder neck reconstruction

8.2.3 Anastomotic Leak

Without leakage, the catheter can be removed on the 5th postoperative day, after retrograde cystography. Earlier catheter removal may be associated with acute urinary retention. A study by Guillonneau et al. (J Urol, 2002; 167:51–56) showed that the risk of acute urinary retention on the 1st day after surgery was 100%, probably due to anastomotic oedema. On days 2, 3 and 4 the risk was 25%, 4.9% and 3.2%, respectively. In our series of the first 900 patients, 19 patients (2.1%) developed urinary retention after catheter removal on days 3–5 after the operation (12 on day 3, 4 on day 4, 3 on day 5). All cases of urinary reten-

tion were successfully treated with 1–4 days of further catheterisation. We routinely remove the catheter on the 5th postoperative day in the absence of leakage.

There is no unanimously accepted method of categorisation of anastomotic leakage in the literature. Even though there are no strictly defined criteria, we have attempted a categorisation facilitating postoperative management of these patients. This classification is based on our scheme of catheter removal on the 5th postoperative day. We routinely perform cystography prior to catheter removal. It must be stressed that the final decision regarding catheter removal is a clinical decision and should not be based strictly upon the recommended classification.

8

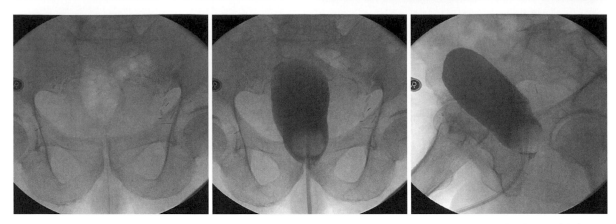

Fig. 8.8. Normal cystogram 5 days postoperatively in a patient with bilateral lymphocele development. Note the elongated deformation of the bladder outline

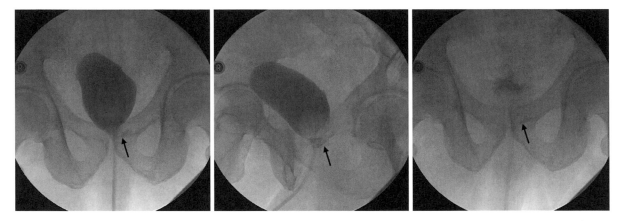

Fig. 8.9. Minor leak requiring an extra 3 days of catheterisation. It has not been proven by clinical studies that such leaks require extra catheterisation time. Nevertheless, it seems to be safest for the patient to wait until the anastomosis is completely water-tight. We initially performed an additional cystography after an extra 3 days of catheterisation but found no evidence of leakage in any patient. We thus decided to stop performing additional cystography in minor leaks

- Minor leak requiring an extra 3 days of catheterisation
- Minor leak requiring an extra 1 week of catheterisation.
- Major leak requiring insertion of mono J catheters and minimum of 2 weeks' catheterisation
- Major leak after dislocation of catheter
- Major leak requiring reintervention

If the urine output through the urethral catheter is less than the output of the drain for more than 48 h, then reintervention and reformation of the anastomosis should be performed. The reintervention is performed endoscopically (laparoscopically). In our series we experienced one such case. We completely opened the anastomosis and performed it again. No further complications were noted. The catheter was removed on the 5th day after the secondary intervention.

Figures 8.6–8.12 show normal cystographic findings as well as the various types of anastomotic leaks.

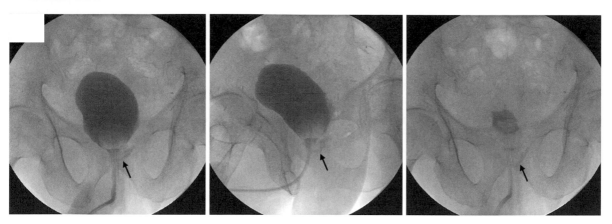

Fig. 8.10. Minor leak requiring an extra week of catheterisation. An additional cystography should be performed before catheter removal. If the leak persists, longer catheterisation time is deemed necessary. In all minor leak patients, there was no urine output from the drain. Antibiotic administration is necessary

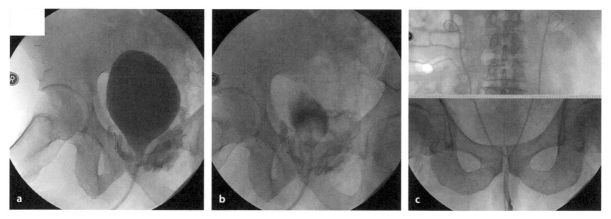

Fig. 8.11. Major leak requiring insertion of mono J catheters. In the case of a major leak, bilateral insertion of ureteral mono J catheters (**c**) should be performed in the effort to keep the bladder and anastomosis as "dry" as possible. The mono J catheters should be fixed to the catheter carefully (suture) and should remain in place for 10–14 days. Cystography should be performed before their removal. The urethral catheter balloon should be inflated with 20 ml to avoid dislocation through the anastomosis

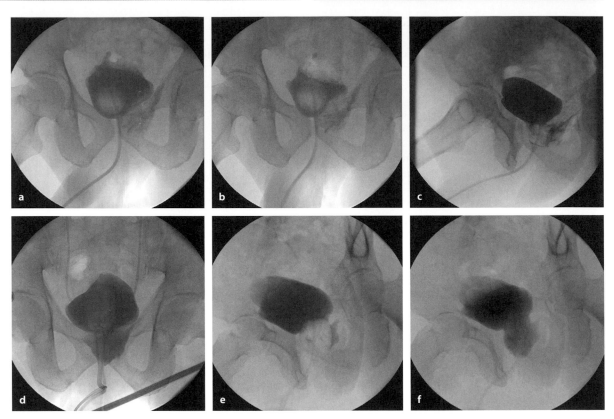

Fig. 8.12. Major leak after dislocation of the catheter. In the case of accidental catheter dislocation (**c**) due to extreme tension of the catheter, a major leak (**a, b**) can be created. This requires insertion of ureteral mono J catheters (**d**). The urethral catheter should be advanced within the bladder and its balloon should be inflated with 20 ml. Both ureteral and urethral catheters should remain in place for a minimum of 2 weeks. These patients will develop a secondary cavity at the site of initial dislocation (**e, f**). The complete healing process of this "additional" cavity can take 1 month or longer. The final cystography (**f**) that is always performed before catheter removal and shows the "abnormal" healing process without any extravasation

8.2.4 Obturator Nerve Injury

The obturator nerve is responsible for the innervation of the medial thigh adductor muscles. Nerve injury is rare and can occur during lymphadenectomy by electrofulguration, complete transection, or entrapment by clips. When electrofulguration is the cause of injury, the symptoms usually subside after 6 weeks. In the case of iatrogenic nerve transection, some authors advocate a microsurgical epineural end-to-end tension-free anastomosis.

In our series we encountered a 0.2% rate of temporary obturator nerve apraxia, treated successfully with neurotropic drugs and physiotherapy. We never experienced complete nerve transection.

8.2.5 Lymphoceles

Lymphoceles occur due to leakage from transected lymphatic vessels. Diagnosis and treatment depend on size, site, and possible infections. Significant lymphoceles may cause pelvic pain as well as voiding problems after catheter removal. Later symptoms can be deep venous thrombosis followed by leg oedema with concomitant pain. A very rare complication is the development of hydronephrosis. Infected lymphoceles are often associated with febrile conditions. Percutaneous drainage, sclerotherapy, or laparoscopic transperitoneal fenestration may be performed.

When a small symptomatic lymphocele is diagnosed by ultrasonography, percutaneous drainage and sclerotherapy can be performed as a first-line treatment, but its success rate is under 50%. The percutaneous drain should be closed for 1 day to evaluate the effect of sclerotherapy treatment. If lymph production continues, a laparoscopic fenestration should be performed.

Patients with infected symptomatic lymphoceles (fever, leucocytosis, increased C reactive protein) are initially treated by percutaneous drainage and antibiotic coverage. Laparoscopic fenestration is performed when the patient has recovered his normal condition.

Access for the fenestration is achieved through the periumbilical trocar (minilaparotomy), the site of previous placement of the laparoscope during the EE-RPE. In contrast to EERPE, lymphocele fenestration requires a transperitoneal approach. In most cases the lymphocele is clearly visible and the fenestration is performed starting ventrally and concluding dorsally, taking care not to injure the ureter or the iliac vein. If the site of lymphatic collection is not evident, methylene blue can be injected percutaneously into the lymphocele with the aid of ultrasonographic guidance, or injected via the percutaneous drainage tube.

8.2.6 Miscellaneous

Rare untoward postoperative events include perineal pain, pubic osteitis, urosepsis, penile haematoma and perineal haematoma. If a perineal haematoma causes voiding disorders, it should be drained under perineal ultrasonographic guidance.

Haemostasis in Radical Prostatectomy

9

Evangelos N. Liatsikos · Paraskevi Katsakiori · Jens-Uwe Stolzenburg

9.1 Introduction

Adequate haemostasis is essential in every surgical procedure. Uncontrolled bleeding hinders the surgeon's work and potentially threatens the patient's life. Particularly, during laparoscopic radical prostatectomy, even small amounts of blood may critically impair the view at a site where vision is already restricted a priori. For this reason, haemostasis in laparoscopic procedures focuses mainly on primary prevention of bleeding.

There are various methods of securing surgical haemostasis, including mechanical means (sutures, ligatures or staples), vessel coagulation (electrocautery or ultrasonic energy) and tissue sealing. Frequently, more than one type of procedure is needed to achieve satisfactory haemostasis. The application of mechanical devices is time consuming, requires good access to the vessels and leaves a foreign material inside the patient, which may lead to complications. Haemostatic clips are utilised for the mechanical ligation of vessels with a diameter of 3–7 mm. Stapling devices are costly for multiple single-vessel applications [1]. Electrocoagulation systems are quickly applied and do not introduce foreign materials. They are capable of sealing vessels with a diameter up to 2–3 mm. However, possible lateral thermal damage and potential tissue necrosis impede their application. In addition, they are unreliable for vessels with a diameter >2 mm [2]. Tissue sealants can be applied with or without clips or staples and are capable of providing satisfactory haemostasis alone or in conjunction with other haemostatic methods.

This chapter provides an overview of the various methods of haemostasis.

9.2 Mechanical Means

Mechanical means of haemostasis include mechanical compression, sutures, clips and staples [3]. The same principles are used in both open and laparoscopic radical prostatectomy. Proper tissue dissection and early identification of the supplying blood vessels, preferably before bleeding occurs, are necessary. Dissection with a laparoscopic styptic stick helps to control bleeding from the adjacent vessels.

Local compression with a sponge in the case of uncontrollable venous bleeding provides the surgeon with time to elaborate further strategies for final haemostasis. Local compression by itself may sometimes be sufficient. If not, the application of tissue sealants in combination with local mechanical compression may adequately seal large vessels, even the vena cava.

Suturing techniques in laparoscopic radical prostatectomy differ from those in open surgery and require advanced laparoscopic skills. Freehand intracorporeal suturing is preferable to external knotting because it avoids excessive traction during suturing. The use of endo-loops may be of great help, particularly for surgeons inexperienced in endoscopic suturing. During the application of endo-loops, however, a significant amount of healthy tissue is sacrificed. Moreover, the loops may slip off due to tissue ischaemia, and loops that remain in place may loosen.

Laparoscopic vascular clips are the preferred tool for sealing blood vessels. Small amounts of bleeding may still occur, however, either due to malposition of clips or because the enclosed bundles of tissue are too small. Titanium clips tend to slip off during further dissection. For this reason, at least two to five clips are needed for safe control of vessels with a diameter of 3 mm.

Vascular endo-staplers with 2.0- to 2.5-mm jaw width and various lengths have been used to achieve safe occlusion of major vessels and vascular pedicles. The modern endo-staplers are bulky instruments that require 12-mm access ports, utilise three lines of staples for safe vascular control and provide the cutting simultaneously. These devices are costly, single-use instruments and require training before use. The laparoscopic surgeon must always use the appropriate vascular jaw width (not the tissue width) and must ensure that the entire vessel is within the stapler line before firing.

9.3 Electrosurgical Tools

Electrosurgery has been widely used in open surgery for obtaining adequate haemostasis. Monopolar electrocautery was the first tool to be adapted for laparoscopic procedures. However, owing to the high risk of thermal injury in the surrounding tissues during the application of electrocautery, new energy sources have been employed. Ultrasonic coagulation systems have been used in radical prostatectomy with better haemostatic effect, less thermal damage and better functional results.

9.3.1 Monopolar Electrocautery

Although monopolar electrocautery provides adequate haemostasis, its use is restricted by potential complications. By limiting the time of application and the maximum current force, the complications can be minimised. Electrical bypass may occur at sites of low impedance or damaged insulation. This is the reason why we do not use any monopolar energy during EE-RPE. The safety of monopolar electrocautery may be secured by active electrode monitoring. In the case of any break in the integrity of the insulation, the instrument is immediately shut off and the monitoring device does not allow activation if the foot pedal is depressed. Another potential drawback is that re-usable scissors may lose their sharpness after extensive use of monopolar current during dissection. This problem can be solved by using single-use scissors blades for re-usable instruments. Modern re-usable instruments are thought to be safer.

A haemostatic monopolar cautery device that has been utilised in handling capillary bleeding is the argon beam coagulator [3]. This device is a monopolar cautery instrument that uses an argon jet to propel blood away from the surgical field. Although it has proved efficacious in control of minor capillary bleeding, argon beam coagulation alone cannot be successfully used for tissue dissection. Additionally, it is not suitable for managing significant bleeding or haemorrhage from larger vessels.

9.3.2 Bipolar Electrocautery

Bipolar electrocautery has been proposed instead of monopolar and bulk clipping in order to obtain adequate haemostasis and safer dissection and to minimise possible thermal injury of adjacent tissues [4, 5]. Bipolar coagulating forceps have already been used during radical retropubic prostatectomy for coagulation of the vascular plexus [6]. Radical prostatectomy always involves a considerable risk of thermal and electrical injury of the neurovascular bundles and the branches of the pelvic plexus. Significant reductions in intraoperative blood loss and in the need for transfusion during or after the operation were described. Furthermore, the visibility was improved, allowing maximal preservation of the urethral length, complete extirpation of all apical prostatic notches and improved application of the nerve-sparing technique

compared to the standard approach. Urogenital function at 14 months after operation was comparable to that with the standard method, assuming that the parasympathetic nerves and the ventral urethral wall did not suffer any negative thermal effect.

9.3.3 The LigaSure Sealing System

The LigaSure vessel-sealing system was developed in 1995. It works by coagulating the walls of the target vessel by means of bipolar energy. The feedback-control mechanism ensures that the adjacent tissues are not charred by overcoagulation. This instrument is effective in sealing vessels with a diameter of 1–7 mm and results in a high burst strength and permanent seal while limiting the lateral thermal damage [7].

The LigaSure system has already been used in open radical prostatectomy for sealing the pelvic lymphatic tissues and for ligating the lateral pedicles (from the base to the apex of the prostate), the puboprostatic ligaments and the dorsal vein complex. Total operation time and the need for blood transfusion were significantly reduced with the use of LigaSure, compared to conventional ligation [7, 8].

The safety of blood vessel control with the LigaSure system has also been demonstrated in a porcine experimental study. The seals created by LigaSure, were stronger than those accomplished with other energy-based ligation methods (ultrasonic coagulation and standard bipolar coagulation). The seals obtained by the application of LigaSure were able to withstand a minimum of three times the normal systolic pressure [9].

9.4 Ultrasonic Energy Device

The piezoelectric ultrasonic energy device (UED – SonoSurg, Olympus; AutoSonix, Tyco; UltraCision, Ethicon) simultaneously excises and coagulates tissue with the application of high-frequency ultrasound. Dissection and cavitation are achieved using frequencies of 23.5 and 55.5 kHz. The UED minimises collateral damage, avoids tissue carbonisation and reduces potential thermal injury compared to monopolar energy sources. Use of the UED is limited to vessels with diameter <4 mm. In larger vessels, adequate haemostasis cannot be achieved with the sole use of a UED. The same problem may occur at the

Santorini plexus [3]. Nevertheless, many groups have used this instrument in laparoscopic radical prostatectomy due to its excellent haemostatic properties.

Heat production is a source of concern, as unintentional thermal injuries may occur whenever dissecting close to neural structures in laparoscopic surgery. In contrast to bipolar energy, a 23.5 and 55.5 kHz ultrasonically activated device minimises macroscopic tissue charring. In addition the heat production is much slower than monopolar electrosurgery.

Owaki et al. found that the blade of the ultrasonic shears becomes hot after use, increasing to 63°C after 3 seconds and 150°C after 30 s. They suggested that contact of the blade with neural structures immediately following use caused recurrent laryngeal nerve injury in their series of patients undergoing endoscopic parathyroid surgery. This is important to note, since the surgeon has no indication of the temperature of the instrument tips while performing laparoscopic surgery, and there is relatively little space for the dissipation of heat [10, 11]. However, the UED is certainly safe when performing a wide-excision EERPE. For example, we have never had problems with rectum or obturator nerve injuries caused by the use of UED. In nerve-sparing procedures the UED should be used more as a dissecting tool than a cutting tool and should not be activated for a long time near the neurovascular bundle. To date there are no clinical human studies comparing the effect of UED and cold scissors dissection during nerve-sparing radical prostatectomy.

9.5 Lasers for Haemostasis

There are no clinical data on the use of laser devices for achieving adequate haemostasis during open or laparoscopic radical prostatectomy. The most common applications of laser in the field of urology are the incision of urethral/ureteral strictures, ablation of superficial transitional cell carcinoma, bladder neck incision, prostate resection and lithotripsy of urinary calculi [13–15]. Laser prostatectomy has emerged as an alternative to the traditional transurethral resection for the treatment of benign prostatic hypertrophy, aiming to significantly reduce blood loss [16].

9.6 Tissue Sealants

Tissue sealants have successfully been used in the management of adequate haemostasis in various operations, with or without sutures and staples. A number of tissue sealants – commercial and noncommercial – are available, including fibrin glues, cyanoacrylates, polymethylmethacrylates and gelatine products [17–21]. Fibrin sealants seem to be the optimal tissue adhesives, since both the adhesive and the degradation products are biocompatible.

9.6.1 Fibrin Glues

The fibrin glues consist of thrombin and fibrinogen, the plasma derivatives at the end of the clotting cascade (Fig. 9.1). Initially, fibrin sealants contained human fibrinogen and bovine thrombin. The use of a nonhuman protein could potentially cause an anaphylactic reaction or development of antibodies against bovine factor V and subsequent cross-reaction with human factor V. Therefore, recent commercial sealants use human thrombin rather than its bovine equivalent. Other key components that a fibrin sealant may contain are fibronectin, factor XIII and aprotinin.

Aprotinin is a natural protease inhibitor, derived from bovine lung, that impedes clot lysis by inhibiting trypsin, plasmin and kallikrein as well as converting plasminogen to plasmin. However, some researchers have suggested that the aprotinin is not only unnecessary for achieving a stable clot but also entails the rare risk of anaphylaxis. Clotting factor XIII is used to cross-link fibrin monomers into polymers, providing a mechanically stable clot resistant to fibrinolysis [22]. It is added to or co-purified with fibrinogen. Factor XIII is a pro-enzyme that is activated by thrombin in the presence of calcium ions. After its activation, the polymerisation of fibrin monomers occurs within 3 min. Fibronectin enhances the migration of fibroblast and fibroblastic growth into areas of fibrin seal application and therefore participates in wound healing. In purified preparations of fibrinogen, however, fibronectin may be absent.

Careful and proper application of the fibrin sealant is needed in order to achieve optimal adhesion. If fibrin sealant is applied to two surfaces for approximation, the surfaces should be brought into contact immediately, before the polymerisation of the agent. If

Fig. 9.1. Physiological pathway to fibrin

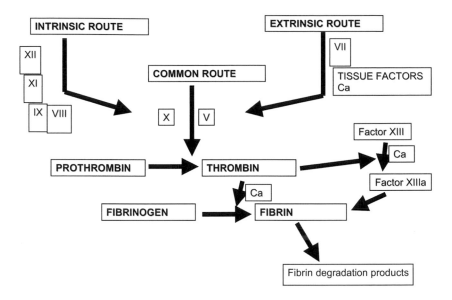

fibrin is applied only to one surface and allowed to polymerise, it acts as an anti-adhesive agent, preventing the adherence of the two surfaces [20]. The two components of the fibrin sealant can be applied sequentially or simultaneously to the surgical field by means of a dual-syringe system – with or without using an endoscopic delivery system –, spraying or sponge application. Commonly, the dual-syringe system enables simultaneous application of equal amounts of fibrinogen and thrombin through a blunt-tipped needle. A long applicator needle with a dual-lumen adapter is available for introducing the agent during laparoscopic procedures. Alternatively, the material can be applied by mixing equal amounts of the two components and spraying with forced sterile gas [20].

To date, fibrin glues have been used for haemostatic or adhesive effect in various urosurgical applications such as kidney-sparing surgery, orchiopexy, pyeloplasty and fistula repair. Their success varies with the depth of the resection and the blood pressure. In radical prostatectomy, fibrin glues have been utilised for obtaining adequate haemostasis with satisfactory results [23–25]. Tissue sealants behave differently in contact with urine. Their adhesive capacity may be reduced because of the fibrinolytic activity of urokinase. Sealants with a lower concentration of aprotinin or sealants containing an antifibrinolytic agent may delay the degradation of the fibrin clot [19].

Another fibrin glue is Tisseel fibrin glue (Baxter, Austria) which contains human fibrinogen, human activated thrombin, calcium chloride solution, bovine aprotinin, fibronectin and factor XIII. When Tisseel initially comes in contact with urine, it tends to maintain a solid form which consequently, turns to a semisolid gelatinous state that is still present at 5 days. Tisseel has been tested in the formation of the urethrovesical anastomosis after radical retropubic prostatectomy [26]. This agent proved to have both haemostatic and tissue adhesive properties.

9.6.2 Haemostatic Gelatine Matrix

FloSeal (Baxter, Germany) is a two-component sealant consisting of a bovine gelatine-based matrix and a bovine-derived thrombin component [27, 28]. The gelatine matrix contains bovine collagen, cross-linked with glutaraldehyde. The matrix can be prepared easily and can be applied in 2 hours. When in contact with normal or sanguineous urine, FloSeal stays in a fine particulate suspension.

The urological application of FloSeal has been described with satisfactory haemostatic results [27, 28]. FloSeal and Gelfoam were used in clipless, cautery-free, nerve-sparing, robotic radical prostatectomy by Ahlering et al. [29]. Intraoperative handling of haemorrhage was satisfactory and only 4 of 17 cases required further management with sutures. No postoperative bleeding events were described.

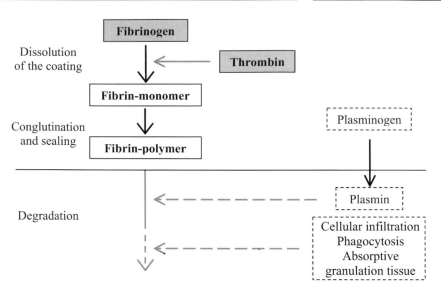

Fig. 9.2. Blood coagulation and degradation of clot and collagen patch. The active components of the TachoSil® coating are shaded

9.6.3 Human Fibrinogen and Thrombin Fleece

The main representative of this category is TachoSil (Nycomed, Austria), a dry, equine fibrin adhesive-coated collagen sponge. Its mechanism of action – like other fibrin glues – is reproduction of the last step of the clotting cascade (Fig. 9.2). It consists of a fixed, solid layer that contains human thrombin and fibrinogen. This layer is anchored on the surface of a collagen carrier. A special fan-like Endo-doc carrier is used to ensure controlled application of the dry fleece.

TachoSil is a further development of Tachocomb and Tachocomb H and differs from them by the absence of bovine aprotinin and by containing purely human coagulation agents. Tachocomb contained human fibrinogen, bovine thrombin and bovine aprotinin, while Tachocomb H contained human fibrinogen and thrombin and bovine aprotinin.

When the coated collagen fleece comes in contact with fluids (e.g. normal saline, body fluids, bleeding surface), the components of the layer dissolve, diffuse into the wound cavities and start to react. The collagen fleece helps to tamponade the wound and therefore keeps the coagulation components in the bleeding area. The required time for gluing is 3–5 min, and during this time the TachoSil must be pressed gently onto the surface of the wound. After its proper application, the sealed surface can be used for further bi-polar coagulation or sutures if needed, without jeopardising the seal. Additionally, TachoSil separates tissues, providing an anti-adhesive effect to the adjacent structures. TachoSil is degraded within weeks or months after its application, either by fibrinolysis and cellular phagocytosis of the fibrin clot or by layer-by-layer degradation of the collagen patch by absorptive granulation tissue, followed by conversion into a pseudocapsule consisting of endogenous connective tissue.

With the use of TachoSil, various vessel or parenchymatic defects can be sealed. A recently published study reviews the application of TachoSil in 408 patients with haemorrhagic risk factors or operations associated with an expected increase of bleeding [30]. The operations were performed on various organs, such as liver, vascular system, heart, spleen, thorax and kidney, and the results supported the efficacy and safety of TachoSil as a haemostatic agent. In addition, when compared to argon beam coagulation, TachoSil proved superior in obtaining effective and fast intraoperative haemostasis during liver resection [31].

During nerve-sparing EERPE in patients with prostate cancer, TachoSil seems to provide adequate haemostasis without jeopardising the clinical outcome. We performed a pilot study evaluating the use of TachoSil during cautery-free EERPE in 20 consecutive patients (unpublished data). The total operative time was 128 min (range 75–210 min). No patient needed blood transfusion or conversion to open surgery. Fourteen of 20 patients were fully continent at 3 months after operation and only one patient needed more than two pads per day. At 6 months, 12 of these 14 men (85.7%) reported full continence and no patient reported needing more than two pads a day. Six out of 20 patients (30%) and 9 out of 15 patients (60%) were potent at 3 and 6 months, respectively. All the patients who reported being potent at 3 months postoperatively were 43–55 years of age. At 6 months, all the patients aged 43–55 years were potent, but only 1 out of 7 (14.3%) aged 56–73 years reported potency. Potency is defined here as a score of 21 points or more on the IIEF-5 questionnaire. The use of TachoSil seems to be safe, as no intra- or postoperative bleeding was reported, and the potency results are very promising.

9.6.4 Experimental Tissue Sealants in Radical Prostatectomy

The use of cyanoacrylates has been restricted due to their rapid degradation to cyanoacetate and formaldehyde, each of which can lead to significant tissue toxicity. This problem led to the development of cyanoacrylates with longer alkyl chains which show slower formation of these toxic products. 2-Octyl-cyanoacrylate (2-OCA) is an agent of this type which is utilised for skin closure. 2-OCA can be used only as a secondary haemostatic factor since it is not able to provide adequate haemostasis by itself. In an experimental canine model, 2-OCA was used in order to form a watertight, vesicourethral anastomosis during open total prostatectomy, with disappointing results [32].

9.6.5 Possible Adverse Events of Tissue Sealants

Tissue sealants have been used in a wide variety of applications over the last 30 years. However, their use has been limited by some potential complications, such as inflammatory or allergic reactions and viral infections [18–21].

Anaphylactic reaction to bovine thrombin is an extremely rare reaction. However, sudden and severe hypotension resulting in death has been reported after application of bovine thrombin to a deep hepatic wound [33]. In most of the recently developed commercial sealants, bovine thrombin has been replaced by human thrombin, avoiding this potential complication. Additionally, allergic reactions have been reported with the use of other nonhuman agents such as aprotinin. The frequency of hypersensitivity to intravenous injection of aprotinin is reported to be approximately 10%.

Bovine thrombin may cause the so-called immunologically induced coagulopathy [34]. In this case, the patient may develop antibodies to plasma proteins in bovine thrombin preparations. Many of these plasma proteins are clotting factors or glycoproteins involved in coagulation. The developed antibodies to these bovine proteins may cross-react with human homologues, leading to significant anticoagulation results.

The possibility of transmission of infection by fibrin sealants has long been a matter of concern and debate [18–20]. Like any other blood product, commercial fibrin sealants bear the theoretical risk of viral transmission. However, no cases of serious viral transmission have been reported since the development of commercial fibrin sealants. Careful donor selection strategies help to decrease viral transmission risk. Additionally, recent advances in viral inactivation technology further reduce the risk of transmission of hepatitis A, B and C and HIV. Various techniques can be applied for viral inactivation,, including vapour heating, steam treatment, pasteurisation, irradiation, solvent detergent extraction and nanofiltration [34].

Finally, caution should be taken during the application of fibrin sealants to avoid the direct injection of the agent into large blood vessels, with the attendant risk of thromboembolic complications. To date, prolonged inflammation has not been reported for fibrin sealants.

References

1. Nelson MT, Nakashima M, Mulvihill SJ (1992) How secure are laparoscopically placed clips? Arch Surg 127:718–720
2. Kennedy JS, Stranahan PL, Taylor KD, Chandler JG (1998) High-burst-strength, feedback-controlled bipolar vessel sealing. Surg Endosc 12:876–878
3. Klingler CH, Remzi M, Marberger M, Janetschek G (2006) Haemostasis in laparoscopy. Eur Urol 50:948–57
4. Chien GW, Mikhail AA, Orvieto MA, Zagaja GP, Sokoloff MH, Brendler CB, Shalhav AL (2005) Modified clipless antegrade nerve preservation in robotic-assisted laparoscopic radical prostatectomy with validated sexual function evaluation. Urology 66:419–423

5. Harrell AG, Kercher KW, Heniford BT (2004) Energy sources in laparoscopy. Semin Laparosc Surg 11;201–209

6. Stief CG (2003) Apical dissection during radical prostatectomy without ligature. World J Urol 21:139–143

7. Daskalopoulos G, Karyotis I, Heretis I, Delakas D (2004) Electrothermal bipolar coagulation for radical prostatectomies and cystectomies: a preliminary case-controlled study. Int Urol Nephrol 36:181–185

8. Sengupta S, Webb DR (2001) Use of a computer-controlled bipolar diathermy system in radical prostatectomies and other open urological surgery. ANZ J Surg 71:538–540

9. Landman J, Kerbl K, Rehman J, Andreoni C, Humphrey PA, Collyer W, Olweny E, Sundaram C, Clayman RV (2003) Evaluation of a vessel sealing system, bipolar electrosurgery, harmonic scalpel, titanium clips, endoscopic gastrointestinal anastomosis vascular staples and sutures for arterial and venous ligation in a porcine model. J Urol 169:697–700

10. Owaki T, Nakano S, Arimura K, Aikou T (2002) The ultrasonic coagulating and cutting system injures nerve function. Endoscopy 34:575–579

11. Ong AM, Su LM, Varkarakis I, Inagaki T, Link RE, Bhayani SB, Patriciu A, Crain B, Walsh PC (2004) Nerve sparing radical prostatectomy: effects of hemostatic energy sources on the recovery of cavernous nerve function in a canine model. J Urol 172:1318–1322

12. Stolzenburg J-U, Truss MC (2003) Technique of laparoscopic (endoscopic) radical prostatectomy. BJU Int 91:749–757

13. Fried NM (2006) Therapeutic applications of lasers in urology: an update. Expert Rev Med Devices 3:81–94

14. Wollin TA, Denstedt JD (1998) The holmium laser in urology. J Clin Laser Med Surg 16:13–20

15. Kabalin JN (1996) Holmium:YAG laser prostatectomy: results of U.S. pilot study. J Endourol 10:453–457

16. Chun SS, Ravzi HA, Denstedt JD (1995) Laser prostatectomy with the holmium: YAG laser. Tech Urol 1:217–221

17. Morikawa T (2001) Tissue sealing. Am J Surg 182:29S–35S

18. MacGillivray TE (2003) Fibrin sealants and glues. J Card Surg 18:480–485

19. Albaba DM (2003) Fibrin sealants in clinical practice. Cardiov Surg 11:5–11

20. Shekarriz B, Stoller ML (2002) The use of fibrin sealant in urology. J Urol 167:1218–1225

21. Schexneider KI (2004) Fibrin sealants in surgical or traumatic hemorrhage. Curr Opin Hematol 11:323–326

22. Buchta C, Hedrich HC, Macher M, Hocker P, Redl H (2005) Biochemical characterization of autologous fibrin sealants produced by Cryoseal and Vivostat in comparison to the homologous fibrin sealant product Tissucol/Tisseel. Biomaterials 26:6233–6241

23. Boeckman WR, Jakse G (1994) Reconstruction of the urethra after radical perineal prostatectomy using fibrin sealing. In: Schlag G, Melchior H, Wallwiener D (ed) Gynecology and obstetrics: Urology, vol 7. Springer, Berlin Heidelberg New York, p 103

24. Lobel B, Ordonez O, Olivo JF, Cipolla B, Milon D, Leveque JM, Guille F (1991) Radical prostatectomy and biologic glue. Prog Urol 1:440–444

25. Patel R, Caruso RP, Taneja S, Stifelman M (2003) Use of fibrin glue and Gelfoam to repair collecting system injuries in a porcine model: implications for the technique of laparoscopic partial nephrectomy. J Endourol 17:799–804

26. Diner EK, Patel SV, Kwart AM (2005) Does fibrin sealant decrease immediate urinary leakage following radical retropubic prostatectomy? J Urol 173:1147–1149

27. User HM, Nadler RB (2003) Applications of FloSeal in nephron-sparing surgery. Urology 62:342–343

28. Richter F, Tullmann ME, Turk I, Deger S, Roigas J, Wille A, Schnorr D (2003) [Improvement of hemostasis in laparoscopic and open partial nephrectomy with gelatine thrombin matrix (FloSeal)]. Urologe A 42:338–346

29. Ahlering TE, Eichel L, Chou D, Skarecky DW (2005) Feasibility study for robotic radical prostatectomy cautery-free neurovascular bundle preservation. Urology 65:994–997

30. Haas S (2006) The use of a surgical patch coated with human coagulation factors in surgical routine: a multicenter postauthorization surveillance. Clin Appl Thromb Hemost 12:445–450

31. Frilling A, Stavrou GA, Mischinger H-J, De Hemptinne B, Rokkjaer M, Klempnauer J, Thorne A, Gloor B, Beckebaum S, Ghaffar MFA, Broelsch CE (2005) Effectiveness of a new carrier-bound fibrin sealant versus argon beamer as haemostatic agent during liver resection: a randomized prospective trial. Langenbecks Arch Surg 390:114–120

32. Grummet JP, Costella AJ, Swanson DA, Stephens C, Cromeens DM (2002) Vesicourethral anastomosis with 2-octyl cyanoacrylate adhesive in an in vivo canine model. Urology 60:935–938

33. Gibble JW, Ness PM (1990) Fibrin sealant: the perfect operative sealant? Transfusion 30:741–747

34. Radosevich M, Goubran HI, Burnouf T (1997) Fibrin sealant: scientific rationale, production methods, properties, and current clinical use. Vox Sang 72:133–143

Extraperitoneal Robotic Radical Prostatectomy: – Operative Technique – Step by Step

Hubert John · Matthew T. Gettman

10

Contents

The extraperitoneal approach for conventional laparoscopic prostatectomy was proposed by Raboy 1997 [1] and popularized by Bollens [2], Hoznek and Abbou [3], Dubernard [4] and Stolzenburg [5]. The feasability of an extraperitoneal access for robotic surgery was reported in 2003 by Gettman and Abbou [6].

The extraperitoneal approach avoids potential small-bowel injuries, allows only a moderate Trendelenburg position and is more comparable to the standard open retropubic radical prostatectomy. This chapter demonstrates step by step the extraperitoneal technique that has been used since 2002 by the first author and performed now in over 400 cases [7]. The transperitoneal access is chosen only after laparoscopic hernia repair with preperitoneal mesh implant, after kidney transplantation or further extensive retroperitoneal surgery.

The access is similar to the technique described in Chap. 7. A short oblique subumbilical incision of 3–4 cm is made. Two Langenbeck retractors expose the anterior rectus fascia, which is incised vertically over a 1 cm length. The retractors are used to split the left-sided muscle fibers of the rectus sheath and expose the posterior rectus fascia and peritoneum. Blunt finger dissection of the retroperitoneal space is performed. In some cases, the tip of the index finger may touch the pubic symphysis during blunt dissection. Balloon dilatation is performed to expose the extraperitoneal space (Tyco®). The balloon is filled 10–15 times until the extraperitoneal space is appropriately created. Balloon dilation must be performed carefully to avoid bladder rupture, which has been known to occur in cases of overdilation. The camera trocar (Ethicon, 12 mm) is then inserted via the subumbilical incision. An inspection of the extraperitoneal space is performed. Under direct vision, the camera can be used to increase the size of the extraperitoneal space by gently sweeping the peritoneal borders to the side and upwards.

10.1 Installation and Robot Connection

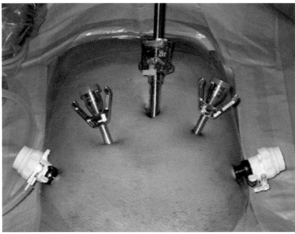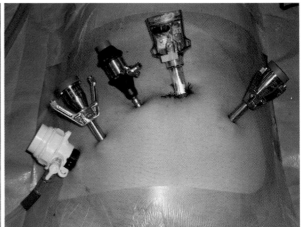

The 8-mm bilateral robot trocars are placed pararectally and two 10-mm standard trocars (Versaport®, Ethicon) just anteromedial of the iliac spine (*left*). In procedures with only one assistant, the left-sided standard 10-mm trocar may be replaced by a 5-mm multiuse trocar, which is positioned between the right-sided robot trocar and the camera (*right*).

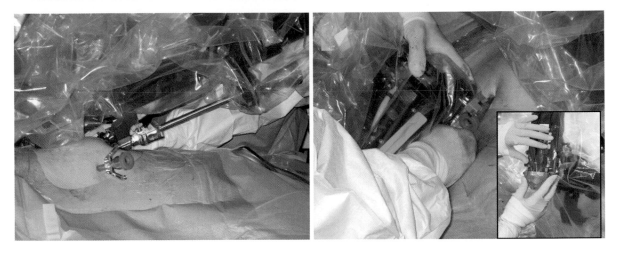

The 0° 3D endocamera is introduced (*left*). The abdominal wall is slightly lifted by the camera arm trocar ("laparo-lift").
The left arm is brought to the left robot trocar and attached (*right*).

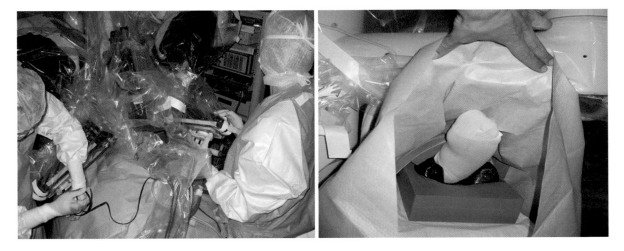

The right arm is also connected and the instruments (bipolar forceps on the left side and round-tip scissors on the right) are inserted under visual control (*left*). The bipolar cable is attached onto the forceps.
Before starting with the operation, always ensure the lower extremities are not compressed by the robotic arms (*right*).

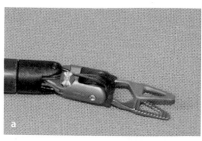
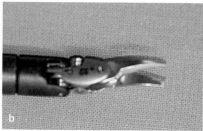
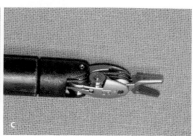

The instruments allow wrist-like instrument movement (Endo-wrist®-technology). We use the bipolar hemostatic forceps (**a**), a round-tip scissors (**b**) and two needle holders (**c**).

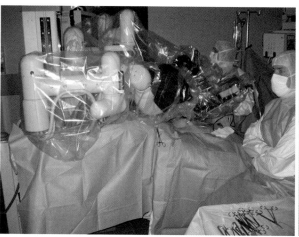
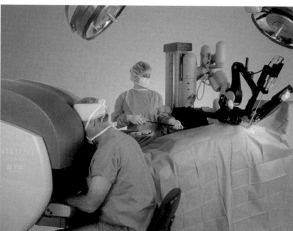

The table-side assistants are comfortably installed (*left*). They assist with an aspirator (right 10-mm trocar), laparoscopic grasper, laparoscopic scissors and clip appliers.

The console surgeon leaves the operating table after port placement and is not sterile scrubbed during radical prostatectomy (*right*).

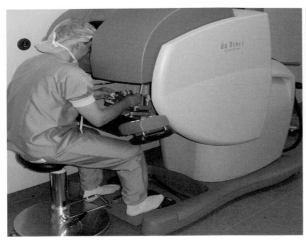 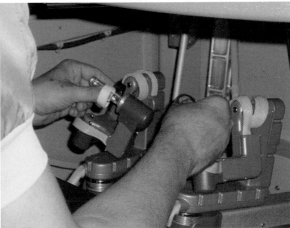

The entire radical prostatectomy is performed by the operating urologist from the remote console (*left*). He controls the robotic arms at the console (camera, working channels, additional fourth arm if installed). The console surgeon controls the interchangeable instruments attached to the two working robotic arms (*right*). They are felt as direct extensions of his arms and fingers.

10.2 Robotic Radical Extraperitoneal Prostatectomy

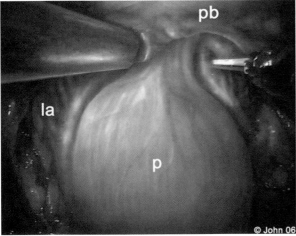 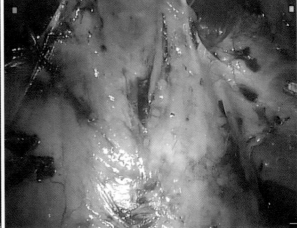

If the preperitoneal space is completely developed, the anterior prostatic surface and the endopelvic fascia are exposed and the fatty tissue overlying these structures is gently swept away.

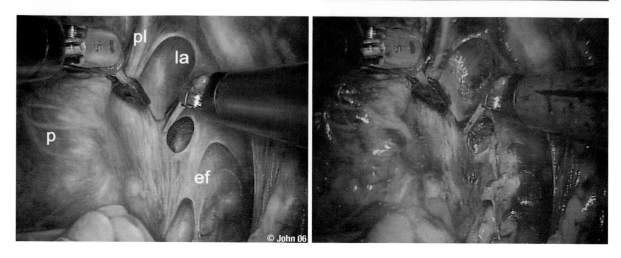

If the endopelvic fascia is freed from the fatty tissue, it is incised from the prostatovesical junction to the apex of the prostate. Fibers of the levator ani muscle are swept off laterally until the entire lateral aspect of the prostate is visible.

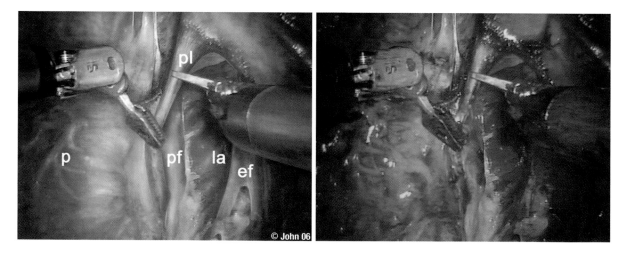

The puboprostatic ligaments are incised to expose the prostatic apex and the urethra.

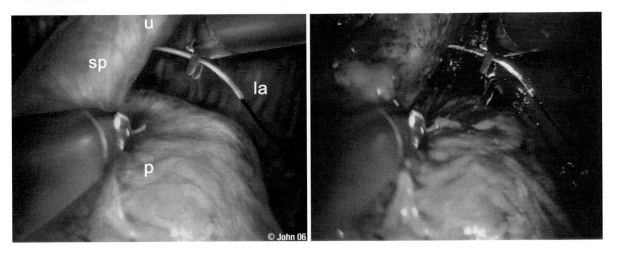

Fibers of the rhabdosphincter are swept distally to the pelvic floor.

Control of the dorsal vein plexus is achieved by a simple or a figure-of-eight ligation. For this we use a 0 Vicryl suture with a slightly straightened MH+ needle.

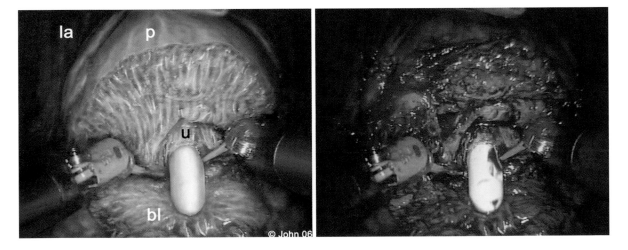

Radical prostatectomy is performed in a descending fashion starting with the incision of the ventral bladder neck. If necessary, the bladder neck can easily be identified by gentle traction on the catheter. The anterior bladder neck is separated from the prostate by blunt and sharp dissection.

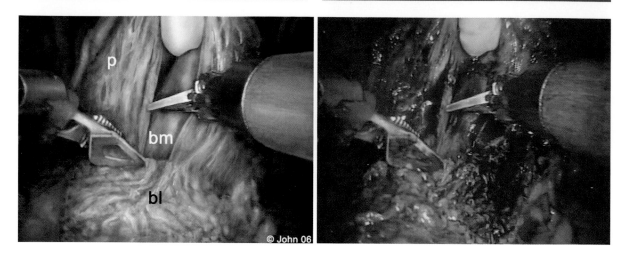

As soon as the urethra is opened, the Foley catheter is grasped by the assistant. Upward traction on the catheter permits the prostate to likewise be rotated upwards and ventrally, thereby optimizing exposure of the dorsal structures.

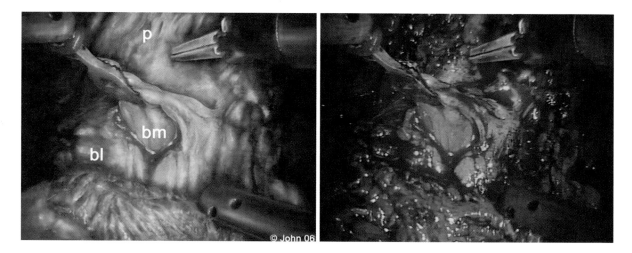

The dorsal bladder neck is incised and the dissection continues in strictly posterior direction until the vas deferens become visible.

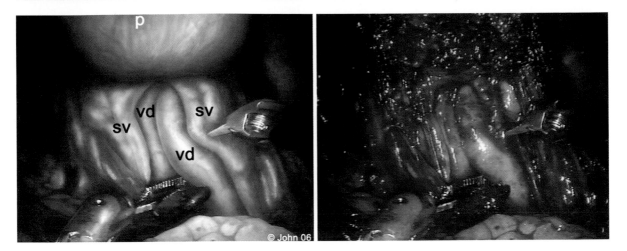

The vasa deferentia are dissected and the seminal vesicles exposed.

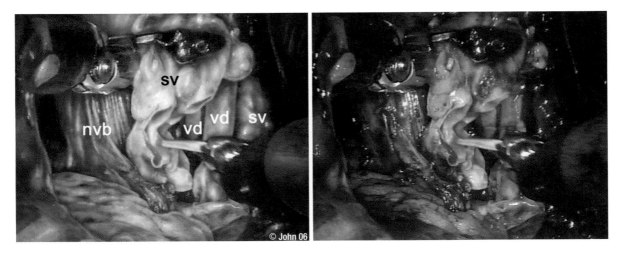

We cut the seminal vesicles leaving their tips in place if PSA is <10 ng/ml and Gleason score <7, in order not to injure the neurovascular bundles, which pass in very close proximity to the seminal vesicle tips and are more likely to be damaged by the added tension that has to be exerted during full dissection of the seminal vesicles [8, 9].

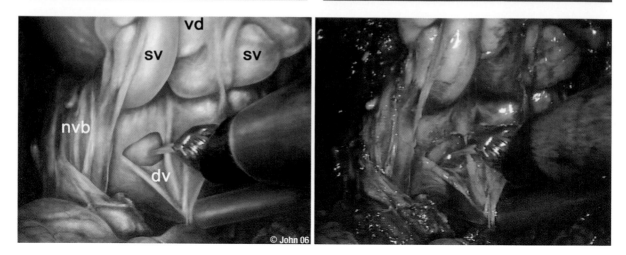

The fascia of Denonvilliers is then opened.

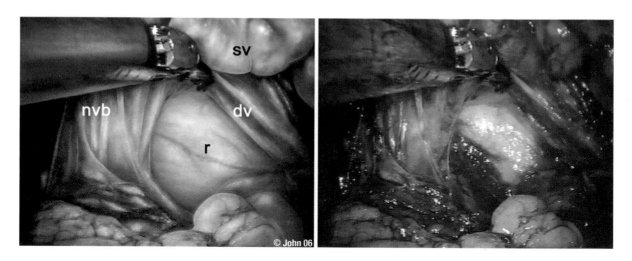

The posterior prostate surface is lifted from the perirectal fat.

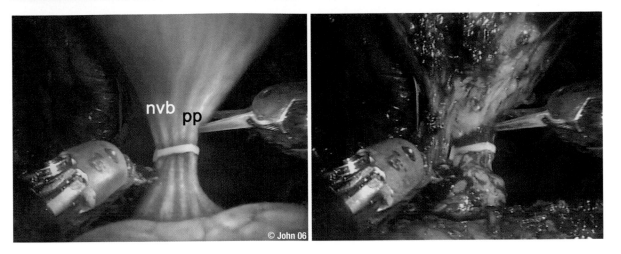

No cautery is used in the further dissection of the prostate along the neurovascular bundles. Hemostasis is achieved by clips if this is necessary.

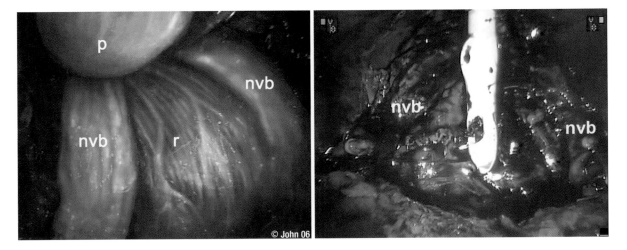

In a nerve-sparing prostatectomy we allow slight bleeding at this stage since it does not interfere with precise preparation and the danger of nerve injury is further reduced. The dissection of the prostate continues in the plane on the periprostatic fascia on both sides towards the apex.

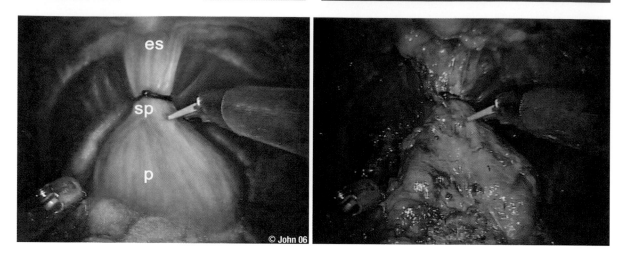

Dissection is continued towards the anterior surface of the prostate. Next, the dorsal vein complex is transected.

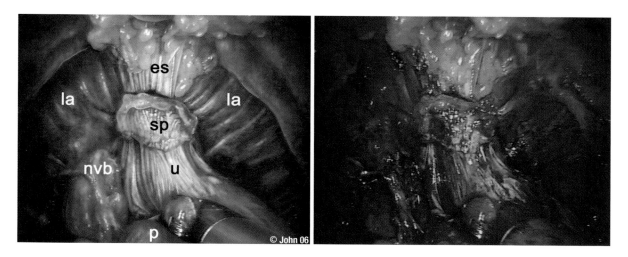

The apex of the prostate is meticulously dissected.

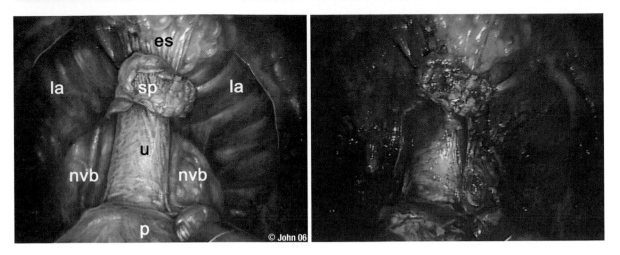

The urethra is exposed and apical prostate tissue retracted to minimize the risk of positive margins.

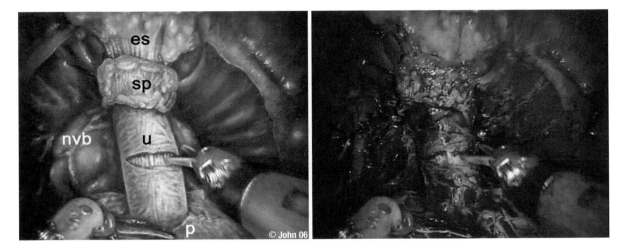

The urethra is opened anteriorly and the catheter becomes visible. The catheter is pulled back into the urethra to facilitate posterior urethral dissection. The rest of the urethra is then transected just distally to the prostatic apex.

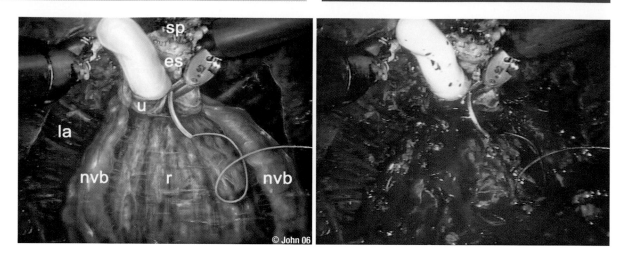

The anastomosis is performed in dorsal to ventral direction, using 2-0 Vicryl sutures with a UR-6 needle.

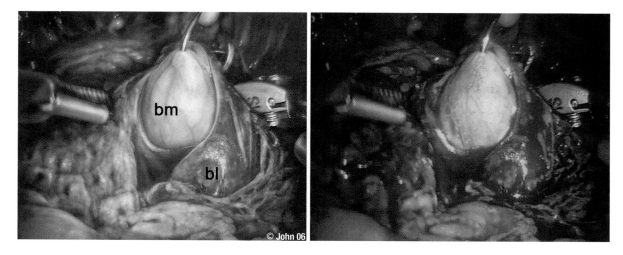

10

The first stitch is placed at the posterior bladder neck. An adequate distance from the bladder neck is warranted to create a stable posterior plate. Care must also be taken, however, to avoid injury to the ureteral orifices.

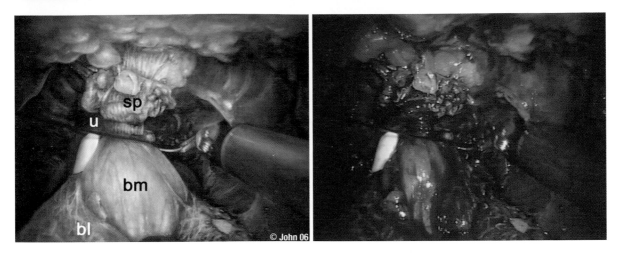

We usually place six to eight interrupted sutures to complete the anastomosis. Before the anastomosis is finished, a 20-F Foley catheter is introduced across the anastomosis and into the bladder. Alternatively, the anastomosis can be performed in similar running fashion using 2-0 Vicryl or Monocryl suture.

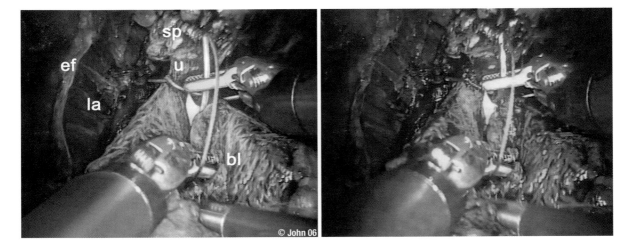

If the bladder neck is widely patent, the bladder neck can be plicated anteriorly with 2-0 Vicryl suture in running fashion.

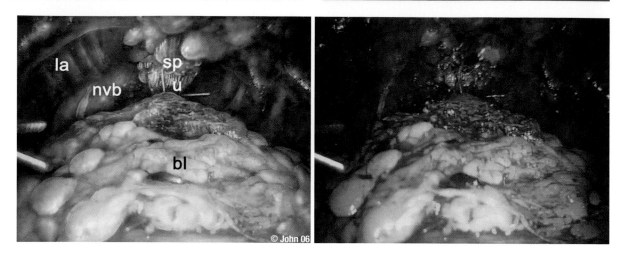

Through the new Foley catheter, 200 ml of saline is filled into the bladder to check the anastomosis for watertightness.

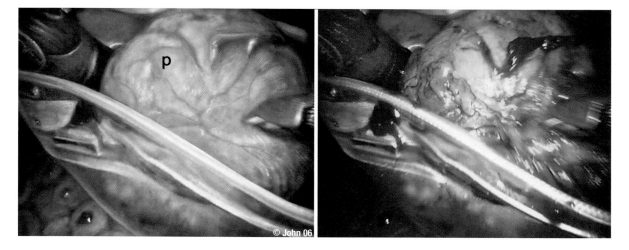

The specimen is placed in a specimen-retrieval bag and extracted through the subumbilical incision. A suction drain is placed through one of the lateral trocars.

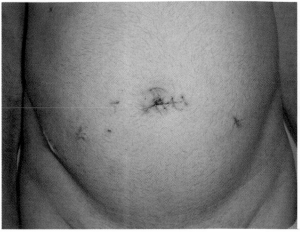 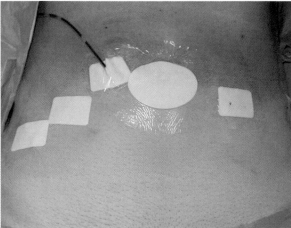

The instruments and the robot are removed. The incisions are closed in two layers. The drainage is removed within 24 h, as is the intravenous access.

References

1. Raboy A, Ferzli G and Albert P (1997) Initial experience with extraperitoneal endoscopic radical retropubic prostatectomy. Urology. 50: 849–53
2. Bollens R, Vanden Bossche M and Roumeguere T (2001) Extraperitoneal laparoscopic radical prostatectomy. Results after 50 cases. Eur Urol. 40: 65–9
3. Hoznek A, Antiphon P, Borkowski T, Gettman MT, Katz R and Salomon L (2003) Assessment of surgical technique and perioperative morbidity associated with extraperitoneal versus transperitoneal laparoscopic radical prostatectomy. Urology. 61: 617–622
4. Dubernard P, Benchetrit S and Chaffange P (2003) Prostatectomie extra-péritoneale rétrograde laparoscopique (P.E.R.L) avec dissection première des bandelettes vasculo-nerveuses érectiles. Technique simplifiée - à propos de 100 cas. Prog Urol. 13: 163–74
5. Stolzenburg JU, Truss MC, Do M, Bekos A, Stief C and Jonas U (2003) Evolution of endoscopic extraperitoneal radical prostatectomy (EERPE)--technical improvements and devlpment of a nerve-sparing, potency-preserving approach. World J Urol. 21: 147–152
6. Gettman MT, Hoznek A, Salomon L, Katz R, Borkowski T, Antiphon P, Lobontiu A and Abbou CC (2003) Laparoscopic radical prostatectomy: description of the extraperitoneal approach using the da Vinci robotic system. J Urol. 170: 416–9
7. John H, Engel N, Brugnolaro C, Muentener M, Strebel R, Schmid DM, Hauri D, Jaeger P (2006) From standard laparoscopic to robotic extraperitoneal prostatectomy: evolution in 350 cases. Eur Urol 5:52
8. John H, Hauri D, Maake C (2003) Impact of seminal vesicle-sparing radical prostatectomy on postoperative serum PSA. BJU Int 92:920–923
9. John H, Hauri D (2000) Seminal vesicle-sparing radical prostatectomy: a novel concept to improve early urinary continence. Urology 55:820–824

The Need for Classification of Complications of Radical Prostatectomy

11

Jens-Uwe Stolzenburg · Paraskevi Katsakiori · Minh Do · Robert Rabenalt · Panagiotis Kalidonis ·
Thilo Schwalenberg · Alan McNeill · Evangelos N. Liatsikos

Contents

11.1 Introduction

Laparoscopic (transperitoneal) radical prostatectomy (LRPE) and endoscopic extraperitoneal radical prostatectomy (EERPE) have been recognised as the standard, first-line therapeutic procedure for the management of localised prostate cancer, especially at experienced centres [1–12]. One of the main quality criteria of a procedure, besides oncological outcome and functional results, is the complication rate.

The literature continuously provides data pertaining to complications, but comparison among series remains subjective due to inconsistency in classification. The absence of consensus among laparoscopists, and surgeons in general, on a common method to report complications has hampered proper evaluation and comparison of different studies. For example, the fenestration of lymphoceles is considered a minor complication by some authors and a major complication by others. How can we compare data if we "speak in different languages"? Proper categorisation of the potential complications after every kind of radical prostatectomy would be of practical benefit for all surgeons. Numerous attempts to categorise complications, their severity, and to create a common objective basis for comparison have taken place [13]. We have previously reviewed the available literature and applied the recently revised Clavien classification as the system for grading complications after radical prostatectomy, including the analysis of our experience from 900 EERPE procedures [14].

11.2 The Clavien Classification System

The Clavien classification system was introduced in 1992 in order to define and classify negative surgical outcomes, which are differentiated by their complications, sequelae and failures. This system was initially used for complications associated with cholecystectomy but it was recently modified and applied to a large cohort of general surgical cases. The modifications from the previous classification consisted of an increase in the number of grades from five to seven, including two subgroups for grades III and IV.

The Clavien system focuses mainly on the necessity of therapeutic management and emphasises the risk and invasiveness of the measures necessary for correction of a complication. Intraoperative complications that are addressed immediately without any deviation from the normal postoperative course of the patient are not graded. Epigastric vessel injury that requires prompt and successful intraoperative correction is an example.

When reporting complications, categorising them as early and late, using 1 month after operation as the cut-off point, is practical, makes their reference easy for all physicians and eliminates eventual discrepancies due to various health system policies. Currently, there is no point in reporting complications as "major" or "minor". The inability of physicians to concur on the definition of these terms results in over- or underestimation of untoward postoperative events. The Clavien grading system, even though it has disadvantages, satisfies the need of standardisation and objectiveness.

11.3 The Grades of the Clavien Classification

In the Clavien classification (Table 11.1), grade I complications include all deviations from the normal postoperative course that do not entail the need for pharmacological treatment or surgical, endoscopic, and radiological intervention. Grade II complications may require pharmacological intervention with drugs that are not administered for grade I complications. Blood transfusions and total parenteral nutrition are also included. Grade III complications require surgical, endoscopic or radiological intervention but are self-limited. They are stratified into grades IIIa, intervention without general anaesthesia, and grade IIIb, intervention requiring general anaesthesia. Life-threatening complications (including central nervous system complications) that require intensive care unit management are classified as grade IVa, single-organ dysfunction, or IVb, multiple-organ dysfunction. Death resulting from complications is classified as grade V. Finally, the suffix "d" is assigned to the respective grade if the patient suffers from a disability at the time of discharge from hospital [15, 16].

Grades I and II of the revised Clavien system correspond to grades I and IIa in the initial classification. Prior grade IIb complications are now ranked as grade III. The length of hospital stay is no longer considered, because there are many differences between countries and medical systems. Life-threatening complications, e.g. acute respiratory distress syndrome with the need for mechanical ventilation, are now ranked as grade IV complications rather than the old

Table 11.1. Clavien classification of surgical complications [16]

Grade	Definition
I	Any deviation from the normal postoperative course without the need for pharmacological treatment or surgical, endoscopic, or radiological interventions. Allowed therapeutic regimens are: antiemetics, antipyretics, analgesics, diuretics, electrolytes and physiotherapy. This grade also includes wound infections opened at the bedside
II	Requiring pharmacological treatment with drugs other than those allowed for grade I complications. Blood transfusions and total parenteral nutrition are also included
III	Requiring surgical, endoscopic or radiological intervention
IIIa	Intervention not under general anaesthesia
IIIb	Intervention under general anaesthesia
IV	Life-threatening complications (including central nervous system complications) requiring intensive care management
IVa	Single-organ dysfunction
IVb	Multiorgan dysfunction
V	Death of patient
Suffix „d"	If the patient suffers from a complication at the time of discharge, the suffix „d" (for disability) is added to the respective grade of complication. This label indicates the need for a follow-up to fully evaluate the complication

grade IIb. Finally, the existence of a complication at the time of discharge is no longer ranked as grade III, but is referred to with the suffix "d".

11.4 Complications of Laparoscopic Transperitoneal and Extraperitoneal Radical Prostatectomy – Literature Review

11.4.1 Transperitoneal Laparoscopic Radical Prostatectomy

Various authors have reported their experience of complications after performing LRPE. Different definitions or classification systems have been used with various results. We now review the recent literature regarding the complications that may occur during or after LRPE as well as their incidence rates.

Dindo et al. defined complications as any deviation from the normal postoperative course, including asymptomatic events such as arrhythmia and atelectases. Sequelae were defined as "after-effects" of surgery that are inherent to the procedure. Neither sequelae nor failure to achieve cure were included in the proposed classification of complications. The main drawback of this classification is the fact that the treatment regimes for a given complication may vary among institutions or countries, thus influencing the ranking [16].

Gonzalgo et al. retrospectively reviewed the records of 250 patients with clinically localised prostate cancer who had undergone transperitoneal LRPE. The updated Clavien classification system was applied for reporting complications. A total of 34 instances of morbidity (13.8%) and zero mortality were noted. A variety of complications were observed, but the majority (94.1%) were self-limited and classified as grade II or III. There were only two grade IV complications (5.9%) and no grade V complications. Postoperative ileus and bleeding requiring transfusion were the most frequent complications, with incidence of 3.3% and 2.8%, respectively. Rectal injuries were recognised in 0.8% of the cases and were repaired intraoperatively without further sequelae [17].

Morbidity, minor and major complications of LRPE were prospectively evaluated by Guillonneau et al. They used the initial classification proposed by Clavien et al. for laparoscopic surgery. The proportion of patients who presented with at least one complication in their series was 17.1%. The major complication rate was 5.3%, comparable with that in other contemporary series. A total of 105 complications were observed in 97 patients (17.1%), including 21 major (3.7%) and 83 minor (14.6%) complications. Reoperation for a postoperative complication was required in 21 patients (3.7%), including 10 (1.76%) who required an intensive care unit stay. In 1.2% of the patients, conversion to conventional retropubic radical prostatectomy was necessary. Mean blood loss was 380±195 ml and the overall transfusion rate was 4.9%. Deep-vein thrombosis occurred in two patients (0.3%) and was associated with another surgical complication but not with pulmonary embolism. Urological, bowel and haemorrhagic complications represented 66.6%, 16.2% and 7.6% (total 89.4%) of all complications, and 20%, 33.3% and 33.3% of all repeat interventions, respectively [13].

Veen et al. used the definition of a complication developed by the Association of Surgeons of the Netherlands. According to this definition, a complication is a condition or event, unfavourable to the patient's health, causing irreversible damage or requiring a change in therapeutic policy, including prolonged hospital stay. Every event resulting in a longer hospital stay, which was a decision of the responsible physician at that moment, was thus registered as a complication. Veen and colleagues did not use a mean duration of prolonged hospital stay as a reference [18].

Bhandari et al. reported their complications of 300 robotic laparoscopic prostatectomies based on the classification of Clavien et al. They characterised these criteria as flexible. Surgeons tend to consider the same complication differently. There were 17 complications, of which 16 (5.3%) were related to surgery and 1 was related to anaesthesia. A total of 11 complications (3.7%) were minor (grade I) and 5 (1.7%) were major (grade II); 3 of these (1%) required reoperation. There were no grade III or IV complications [19].

Arai et al. performed a retrospective evaluation of early complications (within 30 days postoperatively) and postoperative convalescence after LRPE. A 37.2% complication rate was noted (66 complications in 55 patients). Intraoperative complications were reported in 25 of 148 patients (16.9%): ten rectal injuries (6.8%); five bladder injuries (3.4%); five cases of subcutaneous emphysema (3.4%); two intestinal injuries (1.4%); one major vessel injury (0.7%); one ureteral injury (0.7%);

and one obturator nerve injury (0.7%). Sixteen of 148 patients (10.8%) required open conversion or postoperative open surgical repair. The most common postoperative complications were anastomotic leakage (6.8%), wound infection (4.7%) and perineal pain (4.7%) [20].

11.4.2 Extraperitoneal Endoscopic Radical Prostatectomy

As extraperitoneal radical prostatectomy has become a standardised endoscopic procedure, an increasing number of surgeons are embarking upon this treatment modality in various urologic institutions. Therefore, the evolving spectrum of the perioperative morbidity associated with this kind of procedure should be carefully studied. Urologic groups performing laparoscopic radical prostatectomy have documented their perioperative complications but only few have used a standardised classification system [13, 17, 19, 21–26]. The comparison of intra- and postoperative morbidity among the available surgical techniques can be difficult, if not impossible. A common definition and classification of complications among physicians has not yet been established. We now review the current literature on extraperitoneal radical prostatectomy complications.

Bollens et al. reported major complications in 4% of their operated patients. One patient developed an immediate postoperative transient acute renal failure due to tubular necrosis of a solitary kidney and underwent haemodialysis for 10 days. Fortunately, he recovered normal renal function. The second patient developed a postoperative urethrorectal fistula on day 20 which was closed by a perineal surgical approach. Coagulation may have resulted in rectal wall necrosis. Minor complications included three epigastric vessel injuries treated laparoscopically intraoperatively, two urinary tract infections, one prolonged ileus (transperitoneal approach), two urinary leakages (treated by 10 additional days of catheterisation), four transient urinary retentions probably due to early removal of the catheter and treated by 2 days of further catheterisation, one laparoscopic drain removal (transperitoneal approach), one thrombophlebitis and one late hernia at a 10-mm port site (before systematic closure of 10-mm port sites). No other complications such as intraoperative organ injuries were noted, and no death occurred [1].

Recently, Rozet et al. from the Montsouris group reported their results with extraperitoneal radical prostatectomy. No mortality and no cardiac complications were observed. Major postoperative complications occurred in 2% of patients and included pulmonary embolism or oedema, peritonitis and rectourethral fistula secondary to undiagnosed rectal tears, vesicocutaneous fistula, symptomatic lymphocele, urinary retention and anastomotic stenosis in one case each and infected pelvic haematomas and prolonged ileus due to urine diffusion into the peritoneum in two cases each. Of this patient population, 1.7% required reoperation, including colostomy, vesicocutaneous fistula treated with open re-anastomosis, vesicourethral stenosis treated with endoscopic incision, laparoscopic lymphocele marsupialisation and acute urinary retention treated with endoscopic vesical clots evacuation in one case each and infected pelvic haematoma evacuation and endoscopic bilateral ureteral stent placement in two cases each. The incidence of minor complications was 9.2%, representing a total of 55 cases. Anastomotic leaks occurred in 30 cases. Urinary retention following bladder catheter removal was present in 20 patients, requiring new catheter placement for 1 week. Three patients had lymphoceles and two suffered an umbilical port site abscess. Seven blood transfusions (1.2%) with an average of 3 units of packed cells (range 2–6) were also necessary [6].

Martina et al. presented their experience with the extraperitoneal radical prostatectomy of a "laparoscopy-naive" urologist. A total of 16 complications occurred in 114 cases (14%). Half of these complications were early, half late. The early complications were pelvic haematoma in one patient, epigastric vessel haemorrhage in one, transitory anuria in one, urinary retention in four, and gross haematuria in one patient. The epigastric vessel injury was diagnosed in the immediate postoperative period and was treated surgically. It was the only early complication requiring reoperation, resulting in the overall early reoperation rate of 0.9% (1 of 114). No deaths occurred. All late complications were treated endoscopically: seven cases of bladder neck stenosis and one of bladder calculus [27].

11.5 Our Experience with EERPE

Our published experience includes a series of 900 patients who underwent EERPE [14]. The complications of these cases were categorised according to the revised Clavien classification (Table 11.2) [16].

The incidence of intraoperative complications was 0.8%. Six patients (0.7%) sustained intraoperative rectal injuries, which were treated endoscopically with a two-layer suture. In one case (0.1%), injury of the interureteric crest occurred intraoperatively and double pigtail stents were inserted bilaterally to ascertain ureteral viability. The bladder neck was reconstructed at the 6 o'clock position. The placement of the trocar caused intraoperative epigastric vessel injury in nine cases (1%), but this was promptly identified and was managed by coagulation, clipping or suturing. This intraoperative event did not influence the postoperative course of the patients and did not require any further treatment. These patients were not included in the Clavien grading.

Early postoperative reinterventions were necessary in 3.4% of cases: in 8 patients due to bleeding (3× open revision, 5× endoscopic revision), in 2 patients due to postoperative anuria (1× bilateral double J catheter insertion, 1× percutaneous nephrostomy), in 14 patients due to symptomatic lymphoceles (5× percutaneous drainage, 9× laparoscopic fenestrations), in 1 patient with a rectourethral fistula (colostomy, secondary repair), and in 6 patients due to major anastomotic leakage (5× mono J catheter placement, 1× endoscopic performance of a neo-anastomosis during the 2nd postoperative day).

Urinary retention after catheter removal developed in 19 patients on days 3–5 after the operation (12× day 3, 4× day 4, 3× day 5) and was treated with 1–4 days of catheterisation. Such complications have not been reported by laparoscopic or open surgery groups because they tend to remove the catheter later on day 7–8, or even after 14 days. Catheterisation for an additional 2–3 days is considered a complication according to the Clavien system. However, the responsible physician would not accept it as a complication if the overall catheterisation time is shorter than that in other series reported in the literature. In this case the Clavien system fails to take account of differences in medical practice. A report by Guillonneau et al. showed that when removing the catheter on the 2nd, 3rd or 4th day the risk of acute urinary retention is 25%, 4.9% and 3.2%, respectively [13]. We routinely

Table 11.2. Complications of EERPE[a]

Clavien grade	Complication	n (%)	Management
	Intraoperative complications		
I	Rectal injury	6 (0.7%)	Two-layer suture
IIIa	Injury to interureteric crest	1 (0.1%)	DJ catheter placement and suture
	Early complications (<1 month postoperatively)		
I	Urinary retention	19 (2.1%)	1–4 extra days of catheterisation
I"d"	Anastomotic leakage	16 (1.8%)	Prolonged catheterisation (>14 days)
II	Preperitoneal haematoma	1 (0.1%)	Conservative
II	Deep vein thrombosis	6 (0.7%)	Conservative
II	Urinary tract infection	8 (0.9%)	Conservative (antibiotics)
II"d"	Temporary obturator nerve apraxia	2 (0.2%)	Conservative
II"d"	Pubic osteitis	1 (0.1%)	Antibiotic treatment
IIIa	Perineal haematoma	2 (0.2%)	Percutaneous drainage
IIIa	Anuria	2 (0.2%)	DJ catheter placement ×1
			Nephrostomy placement ×1
IIIa	Symptomatic lymphocele	14 (3.6%[b])	Percutaneous puncture ×5
IIIb			Laparoscopic fenestration ×9
IIIa	Anastomotic leakage	6 (0.7%)	Mono J catheter placement ×5
IIIb			Re-anastomosis (2nd postoperative day) ×1
IIIb	Rectourethral fistula	1 (0.1%)	Colostomy, secondary repair
	Bleeding/haematoma	9 (1%)	Endoscopic revision ×4
			Open revision ×5
IVa	Urosepsis	1 (0.1%)	Conservative (intensive care for 5 days)
	Late complications (>1 month postoperatively)		
IIIa	Anastomotic stricture	2 (0.2%)	Endoscopic bladder neck incision
IIIb	Port site hernia	2 (0.2%)	Open repair
IVa	Myocardial infarction	1 (0.1%)	Surgical treatment
IVa	Cerebrovascular event	1 (0.1%)	Conservative

[a] 101 complications in 98 patients out of 900 EERPEs

[b] The occurrence of symptomatic lymphoceles (3.6%) refers to the 389 patients in whom a lymphadenectomy was deemed necessary

remove the catheter on the 5th postoperative day, if the anastomosis is watertight, and seldom encounter problems pertaining to retention.

Minor anastomotic leakage in 16 patients required prolonged catheterisation. In general, there is no standardised definition for „prolonged" catheterisation. We consider 14 days as the cut-off point.

In two cases, temporary obturator nerve apraxia occurred and was treated with neurotropic drugs; two patients developed deep-vein thrombosis that was treated conservatively; two developed perineal haematoma and were treated with percutaneous drainage; one developed preperitoneal haematoma and one osteitis pubis, both treated conservatively; eight presented urinary tract infection and were treated conservatively; and one developed sepsis and was admitted to the intensive care unit for 5 days. Minor penile haematomas requiring no intervention were observed in 14 patients, and asymptomatic lymphocele was detected in 19 patients. These latter complications were not assigned a Clavien grade because they did not alter the postoperative course.

Late postoperative reinterventions were performed in 0.7% of cases: two patients with anastomotic stricture were treated by endoscopic bladder neck incision, and two patients with a port site hernia underwent open hernia repair. Myocardial infarction 2 months postoperatively was diagnosed in one patient. Another patient had a cerebrovascular accident 3 months after operation and recovered without any sequelae.

We should emphasise the occurrence of more than one complication in some patients. Postoperative bleeding requiring endoscopic revision and anastomotic leakage requiring insertion of a mono J catheter happened in the same patient. In another patient, rectal injury took place intraoperatively and a rectourethral fistula was formed, requiring a colostomy postoperatively. One patient presented with preperitoneal haematoma and urinary retention.

The application of the recently revised Clavien classification to rank EERPE complications in the above series resulted in totals of 55, 18, 15, 21, and 3 for groups I, II, IIIa, IIIb and IVa, respectively (Table 11.2).

11.6 Conclusions

Emphasis should be placed on the need for a widely accepted nomenclature and rating of complications. The medical community has not enthusiastically accepted the efforts at classification of complications due to legal and financial considerations and tends to underestimate the importance of reporting complications.

The ideal classification for reporting the complications of any therapeutic procedure must meet many requirements and serve many needs. Web-based platforms developing a document-based global complication database could be of particular interest. Further efforts should be made, with international collaboration, to establish a well-accepted and efficient method for categorising and reporting complications that will assist the surgeon in understanding and resolving clinical problems. In the meantime, the Clavien classification system should be adopted by as many authors as possible to enable correct interpretation and comparison of complications among various series.

References

1. Bollens R, Vanden Bossche M, Roumeguere T, Damoun A, Ekane S, Hoffmann P, Zlotta AR, Schulman CC (2001) Extraperitoneal laparoscopic radical prostatectomy. Results after 50 cases. Eur Urol 40:65–69
2. Cathelineau X, Cahill D, Widmer H, Rozet F, Baumert H, Vallancien G (2004) Transperitoneal or extraperitoneal approach for laparoscopic radical prostatectomy: a false debate over a real challenge. J Urol 171:714–716
3. Rassweiler J, Sentker L, Seemann O, Hatzinger M, Stock C, Frede T (2001) Heilbronn laparoscopic radical prostatectomy. Technique and results after 100 cases. Eur Urol 40:54–64
4. Rassweiler J, Seeman O, Schulze M, Teber D, Hatzinger M, Frede T (2003) Laparoscopic versus open radical prostatectomy: a comparative study at a single institution. J Urol 169:1689–1693
5. Guillonneau B, El-Fettouh H, Baumert H, Cathelineau X, Doublet JD, Fromont G, Vallancien G (2003) Laparoscopic radical prostatectomy: oncological evaluation after 1,000 cases at Montsouris Institute. J Urol 169:1261–1266
6. Rozet F, Galiano M, Cathelineau X, Barret E, Cathala N, Vallancien G (2005) Extraperitoneal laparoscopic radical prostatectomy: a prospective evaluation of 600 cases. J Urol 174:908–911
7. Stolzenburg J-U, Rabenalt R, Do M, Ho K, Dorschner W, Waldkirch E, Jonas U, Schütz A, Horn L, Truss MC (2005) Endoscopic extraperitoneal radical prostatectomy (EERPE) – oncological and functional results after 700 procedures. J Urol 174:1271–1275
8. Stolzenburg J-U, Do M, Rabenalt R, Pfeiffer H, Horn L, Truss MC, Jonas U, Dorschner W (2003) Endoscopic extraperitoneal radical prostatectomy (EERPE) – initial experience after 70 procedures. J Urol 169:2066–2071
9. Stolzenburg J-U, Do M, Pfeiffer H, König F, Aedtner B, Dorschner W (2002) The endoscopic extraperitoneal radical prostatectomy (EERPE): technique and initial experience. World J Urol 20:48–55
10. Stolzenburg J-U, Truss MC (2003) Technique of laparoscopic (endoscopic) radical prostatectomy. BJU Int 91:749–757
11. Stolzenburg J-U, Truss MC, Do M, Rabenalt R, Pfeiffer H, Dunzinger M, Aedtner B, Stief CG, Jonas U, Dorschner W (2003) Evolution of endoscopic extraperitoneal radical prostatectomy (EERPE) – technical improvements and development of a nerve-sparing, potency-preserving approach. World J Urol 21:147–152
12. Stolzenburg J-U, Truss MC, Bekos A, Do M., Rabenalt R, Stief CG, Hoznek A, Abbou CC, Neuhaus J, Dorschner W (2004) Does the extraperitoneal laparoscopic approach improve the outcome of radical prostatectomy? Curr Urol Rep 5:115–122

13. Guillonneau B, Rozet F, Cathelineau X, Lay F, Barret E, Doublet JD, Baumert H, Vallancien G (2002) Perioperative complications of laparoscopic radical prostatectomy: the Montsouris 3-year experience. J Urol 167:51–56

14. Stolzenburg J-U, Rabenalt R, Do M, Lee B, Truss MC, Schaibold H, Burchardt M, Jonas U, Liatsikos EN (2006) Categorisation of complications of endoscopic extraperitoneal and laparoscopic transperitoneal radical prostatectomy. World J Urol 24:88–93

15. Clavien PA, Sanabria JR, Strasberg SM (1992) Proposed classification of complications of surgery with examples of utility in cholecystectomy. Surgery 111:518–526

16. Dindo D, Demartines N, Clavien PA (2004) Classification of surgical complications: a new proposal with evaluation in a cohort of 6336 patients and results of a survey. Ann Surg 240:205–213

17. Gonzalgo ML, Pavlovich CP, Trock BJ, Link RE, Sullivan W, Su LM (2005) Classification and trends of perioperative morbidities following laparoscopic radical prostatectomy. J Urol 174:135–139

18. Veen EJ, Janssen-Heijnen ML, Leenen LP, Roukema JA (2005) The registration of complications in surgery: a learning curve. World J Surg 29:402–409

19. Bhandari A, McIntire L, Kaul SA, Hemal AK, Peabody JO, Menon M (2005) Perioperative complications of robotic radical prostatectomy after the learning curve. J Urol 174:915–918

20. Arai Y, Egawa S, Terachi T, Suzuki K, Gotoh M, Kawakita M, Tanaka M, Terada N, Baba S, Okumura K, Hayami S, Ono Y, Matsuda T, Naito S (2003) Morbidity of laparoscopic radical prostatectomy: summary of early multi-institutional experience in Japan. Int J Urol 10:430–434

21. Hoznek A, Antiphon P, Borkowski T, Gettman M, Katz R, Salomon L, Zaki S, de la Taille A, Abbou CC (2003) Assessment of surgical technique and perioperative morbidity associated with extraperitoneal versus transperitoneal laparoscopic radical prostatectomy. Urology 61:617–622

22. Dillioglugil Ö, Leibman BD, Leibman NS, Kattan MW, Rosas AL, Scardino PT (1997) Risk factors for complications and morbidity after radical retropubic prostatectomy. J Urol 157:1760–1767

23. Guillonneau B, Gupta R, El Fettouh H, Cathelineau X, Baumert H, Vallancien G (2003) Laparoscopic management of rectal injury during radical prostatectomy. J Urol 169:1694–1696

24. Bishoff JT, Allaf ME, Kirkels W, Moore RG, Kavoussi LR, Schroder F (1999) Laparoscopic bowel injury: incidence and clinical presentation. J Urol 161:887–890

25. Vallancien G, Cathelineau X, Baumert H, Doublet JD, Guillonneau B (2002) Complications of transperitoneal laparoscopic surgery in urology: review of 1,311 procedures at a single center. J Urol 168:23–26

26. Van Velthoven RF (2005) Laparoscopic radical prostatectomy: transperitoneal versus retroperitoneal approach: is there an advantage for the patient? Curr Opin Urol 15:83–88

27. Martina GR, Giumelli P, Scuzzarella S, Remotti M, Caruso G, Lovisolo J (2005) Laparoscopic extraperitoneal radical prostatectomy – learning curve of a laparoscopy-naive urologist in a community hospital. Urology 65:959–963

11

Modular Training in Endoscopic Extraperitoneal Radical Prostatectomy

12

Jens-Uwe Stolzenburg · Robert Rabenalt · Minh Do · Michael Truss · Shiv Mohan Bhanot ·
Hartwig Schwaibold · Kossen Ho · Chris Anderson · Alan McNeill · Paraskevi Katsakiori ·
Evangelos N. Liatsikos

Contents

12.1 Introduction

Laparoscopic radical prostatectomy (LRPE) is one of the most technically demanding procedures in urology. However, the development and the standardisation of this technique have reached the point where many institutions no longer offer their patients the choice of open radical prostatectomy [1–6]. Thus one of the main focuses today is to evolve and ameliorate training facilities and establish teaching schemes for laparoscopic procedures in general and especially for this very complex operation.

Teaching operative skills is crucial to urology resident training. The first mentor–trainee model was introduced by Halstead. This model has long been applied for mentoring conventional surgical techniques to residents [7]. The development of the laparoscopic procedure has created new needs that the existing training modalities are unable to fulfil. Procedures are performed under inconvenient conditions, such as a two-dimensional video image, decreased tactile feedback, paradoxical instrument movements, and a limited range of motion [8–11].

In general surgery, laparoscopy is the „gold-standard" treatment option for cholecystectomy and antireflux surgery. Advantages of minimally invasive approaches over conventional open surgery have been demonstrated for a plethora of other operations. There is a consensus among surgeons that laparoscopic procedures of low and intermediate difficulty are part of general surgical training. Procedures such as laparoscopic cholecystectomy and laparoscopic hernia repair belong to the most commonly performed surgical procedures paving the way to the widespread use of laparoscopic techniques in general surgery. In contrast, in urology there are no such high-volume procedures with low or intermediate difficulty. Procedures with a low level of difficulty, e.g. laparoscopic varicocele repair, face competition from other minimally invasive procedures such as the retrograde injection of sclerosing agents or embolisation. This has led to a slower development of laparoscopic procedures in urology.

Despite these difficulties laparoscopic procedures have become part of the standard armamentarium, mostly in urologic centres with a special focus on laparoscopy. However, this development has caused an additional challenge to the urologic community: surgeons in training will have to learn the laparoscopic techniques without having ever performed the procedure in a conventional way.

The task of introducing laparoscopy to resident urologists with no prior training in this type of operation is difficult. Transfer of skills based on techniques learned while performing open surgery is neither appropriate nor effective. A variety of workshops during postgraduate education courses attempt to provide basic skills and more advanced notions of laparoscopic techniques. Colegrove et al. reported that only 54.3% of trainees who attended such courses were able to perform laparoscopic surgery 5 years after the workshop, in contrast to urologists who had received training in a structured and organised laparoscopic fellowship and were performing on average approximately 25 cases per year [12].

12.2 Laparoscopic Simulator Training

The necessity for the creation of laparoscopic courses is obvious. A variety of models have been developed to train residents in basic laparoscopic skills within a structured curriculum, in a controlled environment, and free of the emotional stress of operating on real patients. A plethora of simulators (dry laboratories), ranging from mirrored boxes to expensive virtual-reality computer software, have been claimed to be effective in the acquisition of laparoscopic skills. Despite the usefulness of box trainers in basic laparoscopic skills acquisition, they offer an unrealistic environment. Laparoscopists concur that practicing on simulators improves the skills and facilitates performance in live animals (wet laboratories).

Animal models offer an alternative training system with greater realistic potential. Especially the young pig model (animals 2–5 months old – older pigs are difficult to handle because of their size) offers a wide range of training applications. The similarity of pig and human anatomy constitutes a useful „living model" for amelioration of laparoscopic skills. The trainees can practice a wide range of procedures and deal with their complications „in vivo". The pig model encompasses easy and more demanding tasks. Certainly, the performance of a laparoscopic nephrectomy requires less expertise than the vesicourethral anastomosis during a radical prostatectomy.

Especially considering that the anatomy of animal organs is not absolutely identical to that of humans, we have to accept that animal models are still far from ideal. Nevertheless, training with these models enables mastering of dissection and haemostatic tech-

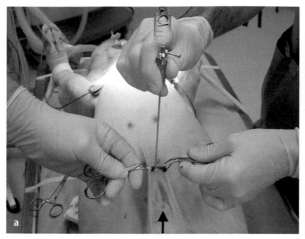

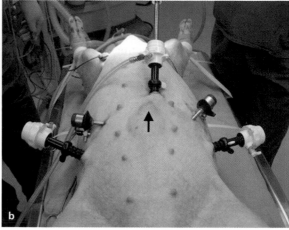

Fig. 12.1. a Positioning of the Veress needle. Note that there is no actual umbilicus in the pig. The arrow marks the penis. Two Backhaus clamps are used to facilitate insertion. b Trocar placement for pelvic surgery in pigs. The position of trocars mimics that of EERPE in human even though only a transperitoneal prostatectomy is possible in pigs

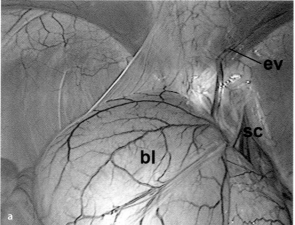

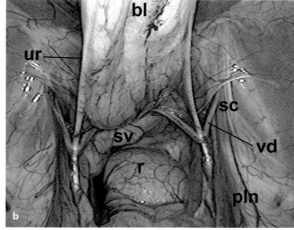

Fig. 12.2. a View into the pelvis of the pig after trocar placement. The bladder should be emptied through a percutaneous puncture or by direct incision of the bladder wall. Urethral catheterisation is almost impossible. b The first exercise is the fixation of the bladder to the abdominal wall to train suturing under live conditions. In this figure fixation has already been performed. This allows easy access to the pelvic lymph nodes and seminal vesicles

niques in pulsating tissue. A dry lab could never offer training in conditions so close to reality [10, 13–19].

Figures 12.1–12.4 show the structured wet lab programme that we follow in our institution during our training courses at the International Training Center of Urologic Laparoscopy in Leipzig.

An alternative to the animal model is the pulsatile organ perfused (POP) trainer (Optimist, Austria)

simulating in vivo conditions. POP trainers are equipped with porcine organ systems and perfused with a red fluid to enhance the realism of organ preparation, dissection and suturing techniques.

Animal models are useful in training novice or intermediate-level laparoscopic trainees. However, the trainers should always consider the risk of trainees forming a false impression of their skills when work-

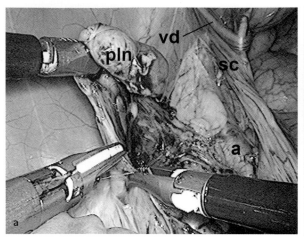

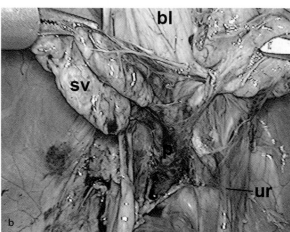

Fig. 12.3. a Pelvic lymphadenectomy. Note that the peritoneal reflection is very thin and there is no retroperitoneal fat. Traction is exerted on the lymph node and dissection is performed with the aid of a SonoSurg device and cold scissors. **b** Freeing the seminal vesicles. As in transperitoneal prostatectomy the procedure starts with freeing of the seminal vesicles after incision of the peritoneum. The dissection should be performed with caution because there are numerous small vessels in the region. Note that the prostate is very small in the young pigs used during the courses (25–35 kg)

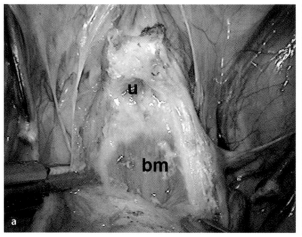

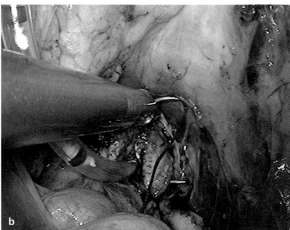

Fig. 12.4 a Anterior bladder neck dissection. The bladder neck dissection starts with a ventral opening of the bladder neck. For training purposes it is more important to have an appropriate urethral stump for the anastomosis than a complete prostate resection. If the trainee does not feel ready to do the entire prostatectomy, an easy exercise is to suture only this ventral incision. **b** Anastomosis. As in humans we start with the posterior part of the anastomosis using a 2–0 Polysorb on a GU-46 needle. A 10-cm segment of a thin connecting infusion line tube is used to guide the stitch at the urethra (it is impossible to catheterise male pigs transurethrally). The ventral part of the anastomosis is performed with the tube in both the urethra and the bladder. In general the anastomosis in pigs tends to be more difficult than in humans due to the small available space in the pig's pelvis. This provides a very good training model

12

ing in wet laboratories [20]. There is no concurrence regarding the necessity to demonstrate the effectiveness of laparoscopic simulator training on live surgery performance [14–19].

Virtual-reality simulation systems for laparoscopy training are continuously reported in the literature. Reproduction of a fully realistic image is impossible due to technical limitations, restricting their use in training processes [13, 17–19].

The ideal way of mastering laparoscopic techniques in vivo is a well-structured mentor-based training scheme [13, 21–24].

12.3 Mentor-based Training Programmes

Mentor-based training seems to be the most efficient way of mastering advanced laparoscopic procedures. Various training programmes have been proposed. Fabrizio et al. proposed the mentor-initiated approach. An experienced surgeon serves as mentor and performs a series of consecutive operations with the trainee acting as assistant. When enough confidence has been gained, subsequent procedures are performed by the trainee with the assistance of the mentor [22]. Bollens et al. suggested a different method. Initial dry lab training precedes assistance in at least 25 cases. A few steps of prostatic dissection are enough for the trainee to accomplish a solo LRPE in less than 5 h from skin to skin. After the first ten independently performed procedures, a visit to the centre of excellence seems necessary to resolve further problems [13]. Chou et al. suggested a mini-fellowship programme during which each participant has 5 days of laparoscopic training, starting with 2 days of laboratory experience under the guidance of an instructor. The next 2 days are completed in operating room and didactic sessions. During the final day, a laparoscopic clinical procedure is performed by the proctor at their home institution [25].

12.4 The Modular Training Programme

An important issue is whether LRPE or EERPE can serve as a training tool for urological surgeons and centres to acquire laparoscopic skills without endangering patient safety and functional results. Furthermore, we need to clarify whether the trainee needs previous open or laparoscopic experience before starting with LRPE or EERPE. The answer to these questions is of paramount importance.

To master these problems we developed a „modular surgical training" scheme which used individual steps of EERPE for resident training. The „modular surgical training" is based on maximised standardisation of the technique of EERPE [26–28]. We divided the entire procedure into 12 individual steps of differing complexity. The levels of difficulty were labelled „modules" (Table 12.1) and graded according to their requisite skills from module 1 (lowest level of difficulty) to module 5 (highest level).

During the learning phase of this operation, EERPE is performed as a three-surgeon procedure with one trainee as first assistant and one as camera operator. It is common for a trainee to begin by holding the camera while gaining basic familiarity with the steps of the operation, before graduating to first assistant. The first assistant is trained in the individual steps of the procedure according to the modular system in a stepwise fashion, with the mentor completing the more difficult steps of the operation. Only when the trainee has satisfied the mentor that he has mastered each module can he progress to learn the next operative step. This stepwise programme of training continues until the trainee is capable of performing the whole operation independently and ensures that the training does not have excessive impact on the overall operation time. As an adjunct to the operative training, daily practice on a „pelvi-trainer" is recommended for suturing practice.

A good example of this kind of tutoring is the urethrovesical anastomosis, which we carry out using interrupted sutures. As in most described surgical techniques for any kind of anastomosis, we start with the dorsal circumference. These stitches are the most difficult ones. The mounting of the needle has to be changed between forehand for the bladder neck and backhand for the urethra. Furthermore, the ureteral orifices can be located very close to the margin at the bladder neck. Hence the mentor would perform the dorsal 4, 5, 6, 7 and 8 o'clock stitches, which are classified as module IV. Then the trainee would take over and perform the stitches at 3 and 9 o'clock, which are the easiest of the anastomotic sutures (module II). The mentor would finish the anastomosis with closure of the bladder neck and the 11 and 1 o'clock stitches, which are generally more difficult (module III). This schedule would be repeated during every training operation, until the trainee had developed

Table 12.1. Modular surgical training: The 12 segments of Endoscopic Eextraperitoneal Radical Prostatectomy, with 5 levels of difficulty. (from 23)

Step no.	Description of surgical procedure	Module (level of difficulty)				
		I	II	III	IV	V
1	Trocar placement and dissection of preperitoneal space	X				
2	Pelvic lymphadenectomy		X			
3	Incision of endopelvic fascia and dissection of puboprostatic ligaments	X				
4	Santorini plexus ligation			X		
5	Anterior and lateral bladder neck dissection		X			
	Dorsal bladder neck dissection			X		
6	Dissection and division of vasa deferentia			X		
7	Dissection of seminal vesicles			X		
8	Incision of posterior Denonvilliers' fascia, mobilisation of dorsal surface of prostate from rectum			X		
9	Dissection of prostatic pedicles			X		
10	Nerve-sparing procedure					X
11	Apical dissection				X	
12	Urethrovesical anastomosis					
	Dorsal circumference (4, 5, 6, 7, 8 o'clock stitches)				X	
	The 3 and 9 o'clock stitches		X			
	Bladder neck closure and 11 and 1 o'clock stitches			X		

12

the requisite skills to progress to modules III and IV in the anastomosis without the help of the mentor.

The aim of two recently published studies was to establish whether the proposed training methodology would ascertain the safe and efficacious training of surgeons with varied experience [20, 29]. Four trainees with varying degrees of surgical experience took part in these studies. After a phase of assisting and camera holding during EERPE, the trainees entered the modular training programme. They required between 32 and 43 procedures within the programme until they were considered competent to perform EERPE without the mentor. An analysis of the first 25–50 procedures performed independently by the trainee revealed mean operative times between 176 and 193 min and a transfusion rate of 1.3%. Rates of intra- and postoperative complications were low [29].

Two of these four residents had no previous surgical experience with open pelvic surgery. Both attended at least one dry-lab course before they began the programme. Previous laparoscopic experience ranged from five varicocelectomies (trainee I) to 80 proce-

dures performed as the main surgeon (trainee II). In a second study, the first 50 and consequent 100 cases performed independently by the residents were compared to the first 50 and last 100 cases (cases 521–621) performed by the mentor [20]. The initial 50 procedures performed completely independently by the residents had mean operative times of 176 and 173 minutes. There were two intraoperative rectal injuries (one patient developed recto-urethral fistula), and 1 haemorrhage and 1 lymphocele postoperatively. The positive margin rate for pT2 disease was 14.3 and 11.5%, and for pT3 tumours 38.8 and 29.1%, respectively. After an additional 100 procedures operated by the same residents, mean operative times were 142 and 146 min. There was one patient who needed a transfusion. Postoperative complications requiring re-intervention were one haemorrhage, two anastomotic leakages and four symptomatic lymphoceles. The positive margin rate for pT2 disease was 12.8% and 6.5%, and for pT3 tumours 33.3% and 26.3% respectively. No statistically significant differences were observed between the residents' and the mentors cases. It was thus documented that previous experience in open or laparoscopic surgery did not affect the performance of the trainees learning EERPE in this programme.

12.5 The Learning Curve for Minimally Invasive Radical Prostatectomy

The number of procedures required to complete the learning curve and ascertain the safe and effective practice of advanced laparoscopic procedures is still into consideration. Although the learning curve for LRPE has been estimated at 40–100 cases, it has been shown that surgeons continue to improve in terms of operative time even after 300 cases [23]. The adherence to numerical values is surely of minor importance. Tang et al. have shown that the training in laparoscopic skills should be more flexible and individualised. The innate ability for manipulative work varies amongst trainees, and some will achieve competence faster than others [10]. It is expected that the conceptual knowledge and manual skill varies among the trainees.

The laparoscopy guidelines of the EAU (2002) support the concept that 50 laparoscopic procedures are required before a plateau in the incidence of complications is reached. It is therefore suggested that only then should an individual surgeon regard himself competent in laparoscopy. In the UK the Endourological Society requires at least 40 laparoscopic procedures to be undertaken or assisted in a 1-year period for a fellowship to be recognised [30]. However, the number of cases is always relative and depends upon numerous factors, e.g. minor or major surgery; role as assistant or first operator; surgery performed independently or with major help from mentor; regular spacing or all cases performed in 1–2 months.

In general, it seems to be problematic to require a certain overall number of laparoscopic procedures for certification. Instead, a defined number of procedures per indication seems more realistic and helpful, especially in procedures of intermediate and high complexity. It is clear that 50 laparoscopic varicocele repairs do not qualify a surgeon for laparoscopic prostatectomy or cystectomy.

Urology residents should be exposed early to high-volume laparoscopic operations (nephrectomy, radical prostatectomy). These operations and training programmes should be concentrated in high-volume centres of excellence in laparoscopy since individual learning curves cannot be mastered in a low-volume setting (i.e. 10–30 prostatectomies/nephrectomies per year). The main goal should be the standardisation of these daily (or weekly) performed operative procedures as well as educational „modular training programmes" in order to shorten individual learning curves and generate common quality standards.

12.6 Conclusions

A highly standardised technique combined with a modular training programme provides a feasible, safe and effective way to teach EERPE. A short learning curve is possible, regardless of the trainee's experience in open pelvic surgery. Although training residents is of paramount importance to the future of urology, it cannot come at the expense of patient safety. Therefore, the main advantage of our modular training proposal is that it provides training in a highly complex laparoscopic procedure without putting patients at risk.

Another fundamental advantage of the modular concept is that the traditional routine of the trainer spending very many hours patiently with the trainee is overcome. In a high-volume centre (more than 200 cases per year) more than one mentor is allowed to train the new trainees. More experienced trainees can mentor the novice trainees in the easier modules. Furthermore, the modular concept also allows for preliminary training in the less complicated modules to be performed remotely from the high-volume centre (multi-centre training). This creates a particularly attractive possibility for training surgeons in a setting where mentors are few, numbers of cases for radical prostatectomy per urology unit are small, and consultant commitments and service obligations make it almost impossible to travel to other hospitals to teach. Provided that the steps of the procedure stay the same and the volunteer mentor is committed to adhere strictly to the standardised technique, there is the opportunity for surgeons to start learning this procedure (easier modules) in a local environment. The final steps (more difficult modules) can then be learned during a substantially shortened fellowship at a high-volume centre.

Figure 12.5 outlines the recommendations for training and implementation of laparoscopic/endoscopic radical prostatectomy in a local hospital. It

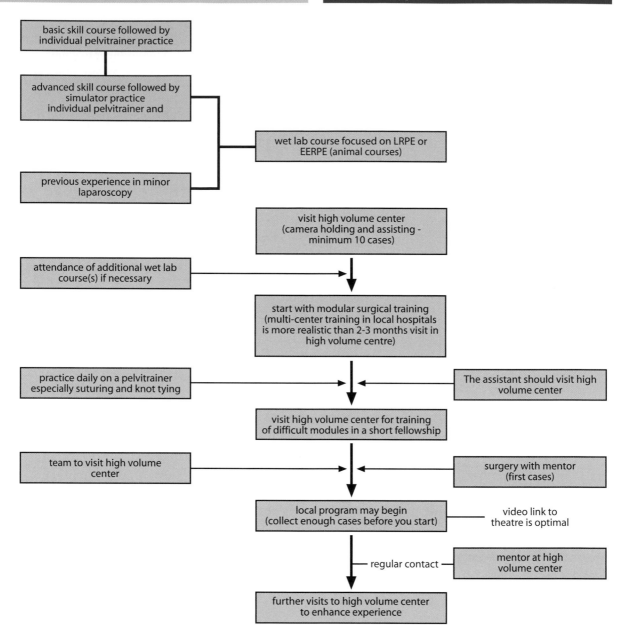

Fig. 12.5. Suggested scheme for training and implementation of laparoscopic or endoscopic radical prostatectomy

must be stressed that when setting up an advanced laparoscopy service the support and encouragement of colleagues, anaesthetic, nursing and theatre staff is essential. A good assistant facilitates the operation greatly, as do theatre nurses who are familiar with the procedure. This can most easily be achieved if the assistant and theatre nurses also spend a period of time at a high-volume centre specifically for training and familiarisation with the procedures, respectively.

References

1. Guillonneau B, Vallancien G (1999) Laparoscopic radical prostatectomy: initial experience and preliminary assessment after 65 operations. Prostate 39:71–75
2. Rassweiler J, Sentker L, Seemann O, Hatzinger M, Stock C, Frede T (2001) Heilbronn laparoscopic prostatectomy: technique and results after 100 cases. Eur Urol 40:54–64
3. Abbou CC, Salomon L, Hoznek A, Antiphon P, Cicco A, Saint F, Alame W, Bellot J, Chopin DK (2000) Laparoscopic radical prostatectomy: preliminary results. Urology 55:630–634
4. Salomon L, Sebe P, De la Taille A, Vordos D, Hoznek A, Yiou R, Chopin D, Abbou CC (2004) Open versus laparoscopic radical prostatectomy: part I. BJU Int 94:238–243
5. Salomon L, Sebe P, De La Taille A, Vordos D, Hoznek A, Yiou R, Chopin D, Abbou CC (2004) Open versus laparoscopic radical prostatectomy: part II. BJU Int 94:244–250
6. Rhee HK, Tuerk IA (2004) Radical nerve-sparing laparoscopic prostatectomy. BJU Int 94:449–474
7. Barnes RW, Lang NP, Whitesede MF (1989) Halstedian technique revisited: innovations in teaching surgical skills. Ann Surg 210:118–121
8. Ahlberg G, Kruuna O, Leijonmarck CE, Ovaska J, Rosseland A, Sandbu R, Strömberg C, Arvidsson D (2005) Is the learning curve for laparoscopic fundoplication determined by the teacher or the pupil? Am J Surg 189:184–189
9. Buchmann P, Dincler S (2005) Learning curve – calculation and value in laparoscopic surgery. Therap Umschau 62:69–75
10. Tang B, Hanna GB, Cuschieri A (2005) Analysis of errors enacted by surgical trainees during skills training courses. Surgery 138:14–20
11. Dagash H, Chowdhury M, Pierro A (2003) When can I be proficient in laparoscopic surgery? A systematic review of the evidence. J Ped Surg 5:720–724
12. Colegrove PM, Winfield HN, Donovan JF Jr, See WA (1999) Laparoscopic practice patterns among North American urologists 5 years after formal training. J Urol 161:881–886
13. Bollens R, Sandhu S, Roumeguere T, Quackels T, Schulman C (2005) Laparoscopic radical prostatectomy: the learning curve. Curr Opin Urol 15:79–82
14. Teber D, Dekel Y, Frede T, Klein J, Rassweiler J (2005) The Heilbronn laparoscopic training program for laparoscopic suturing: concept and validation. J Endourol 19:230–238
15. Nadu A, Olsson LE, Abbou CC (2003) Simple model for training in the laparoscopic vesicourethral running anastomosis. J Endourol 17:481–484
16. Grantcharov TP, Bardram L, Funch-Jensen P, Rosenberg J (2003) Learning curves and impact of previous operative experience on performance on a virtual reality simulator to test laparoscopic surgical skills. Am J Surg 185:146–149
17. Brunner WC, Korndorffer JR, Sierra R, Massarweh NN, Dunne JB, Yau CL, Scott DJ (2004) Laparoscopic virtual reality training: Are 30 repetitions enough? J Surg Res 122:150–156
18. Katz R, Hoznek A, Salomon L, Antiphon P, de la Taille A, Abbou CC (2005) Skill assessment of urological laparoscopic surgeons: Can criterion levels of surgical performance be determined using the pelvic box trainer? Eur Urol 47:482–487
19. Lehmann KS, Ritz JP, Maass H, Cakmak HK, Kuehnapfel UG, Germer CT, Bretthauer G, Buhr HJ (2005) A prospective randomized study to test the transfer of basic psychomotor skills from virtual reality to physical reality in a comparable training setting. Ann Surg 241:442–449
20. Stolzenburg JU, Rabenalt R, Do M, Horn LC, Liatsikos EN (2006) Modular training for residents with no prior experience with open pelvic surgery in endoscopic extraperitoneal radical prostatectomy. Eur Urol 49:491–500
21. Frede T, Erdogru T, Zukosky D, Gulkesen H, Teber D, Rassweiler J (2005) Comparison of training modalities for performing laparoscopic radical prostatectomy: experience with 1,000 patients. J Urol 174:673–678
22. Fabrizio MD, Tuerk I, Schellhammer PF (2003) Laparoscopic radical prostatectomy: decreasing the learning curve using a mentor initiated approach. J Urol 196:2063–2065
23. Martina GR, Giumelli P, Scuzzarella S, Remotti M, Caruso G, Lovisolo J (2005) Laparoscopic extraperitoneal radical prostatectomy – learning curve of a laparoscopy-naïve urologist in a community hospital. Urology 65:959–963
24. Baumert H, Fromont G, Rosa JA, Cahill D, Cathelineau X, Vallancien G (2004) Impact of learning curve in laparoscopic radical prostatectomy on margin status: prospective study of first 100 procedures performed by one surgeon. J Endourol 18:173–176
25. Chou DS, Abdelshehid CS, Uribe CA, Khonsari SS, Eichel L, Boker JR, Shanberg AM, Ahlering TE, Clayman RV, McDougall EM (2005) Initial impact of a dedicated postgraduate laparoscopic mini-residency on clinical practice patterns. J Endourol 19:360–365
26. Stolzenburg JU, Do M, Pfeiffer H, Konig F, Aedtner B, Dorschner W (2002) The endoscopic extraperitoneal radical prostatectomy (EERPE): technique and initial experience. World J Urol 20:48–55
27. Stolzenburg JU, Truss MC, Do M, Rabenalt R, Pfeiffer H, Dunzinger M, Aedtner B, Stief CG, Jonas U, Dorschner W (2003) Evolution of endoscopic extraperitoneal radical prostatectomy (EERPE) – technical improvements and development of a nerve-sparing, potency-preserving approach. World J Urol 21:147–152
28. Stolzenburg JU, Rabenalt R, Tannapfel A, Liatsikos EN (2006) Intrafascial nerve-sparing endoscopic extraperitoneal radical prostatectomy. Urology 67:17–21
29. Stolzenburg JU, Schwainbold H, Bhanot SM, Rabenalt R, Do M, Truss M, Ho K, Anderson C (2005) Modular surgical training for endoscopic extraperitoneal radical prostatectomy. BJU Int 96:1022–1027
30. Bariol SV, Tolley DA (2004) Training and mentoring in urology: the "Lap" generation.BJU Int 93:913–914

Postoperative Management

13

Contents

Inpatient Rehabilitation of Post-Prostatectomy Incontinence

13.1

S. Hoffmann · W. Hoffmann · U. Otto

Although several improvements in the surgical treatment of prostate cancer have been introduced in recent decades, urinary incontinence is still one of the main conditions impacting quality of life after radical prostatectomy, ranking higher than erectile dysfunction [30], at least in the first year.

Besides the postoperative impairments and disabilities, i.e. erectile dysfunction, psycho-physical distress and other postsurgical complications (wound and urinary tract infection, lymphoceles) one important issue in inpatient rehabilitation is postoperative incontinence.

Post-prostatectomy incontinence is mainly caused by sphincter incompetence, in some cases accompanied by overactive bladder, or decreased contractility, but many other factors are involved, e.g. preservation of the neurovascular bundle, age and comorbidity, volume of the prostate, previous transurethral radical prostatectomy (TUR-P), preoperative radiotherapy, spinal cord lesion, urethral stricture, Parkinson's disease, dementia and medications.

The continence rates 1 year after surgery vary between 33% and 100%, depending on the definition of continence (see Table 13.1.1).

Table 13.1.1. Continence rates after radical prostatectomy according to definition of continence

Authors	Year	Number of patients	Definition 1	Definition 2	Definition 3	Surgery
Kielb et al. [15]	2001	90	76.0%		99.0%	RRP
Sebesta et al. [30]	2002	675	43.7%	69.2%	82.2%	RRP
Lepor and Kaci [18]	2004	92	44.6%		94.6%	RRP
Olsson et al. [22]	2001	115	56.8%	78.4%	100.0%	LRP
Madalinska et al. [20]	2001	107	33.0%	65.0%		RRP
Deliveliotis et al. [4]	2002	149		92.6%		RPP
Harris [9]	2003	508		96.0%		RPP
Maffezzini et al. [21]	2003	300		88.8%		RRP
Wille et al. [35]	2003	83		74.7%	88.0%	RRP+/-Rx
Ruiz-Deya et al. [29]	2001	200			93.0%	RPP
Augustin et al. [3]	2002	368			87.5%	RRP
Rassweiler et al. [27]	2003	219			89.9%	RRP
Rassweiler et al. [27]	2003	219			90.3%	LRP
Stolzenburg et al. [31]	2005	700	92%			EERPE

Definition 1: total control without any pad or leakage; definition 2: no pad a day but a few drops of urine; definition 3: one or no pad per day

RRP, radical retropubic prostatectomy; RPP, radical perineal prostatectomy; LRP, laparoscopic radical prostatectomy; EERPE, endoscopic extraperitoneal radical prostatectomy; Rx, radiotherapy

13.1.1 Elements of Therapy

Conservative lower urinary tract rehabilitation is defined as non-surgical, non-pharmacological treatment for lower urinary tract function and includes:

- Pelvic floor training, defined as repetitive, selective voluntary contraction and relaxation of specific pelvic floor muscles
- Biofeedback, the technique by which information about a normally unconscious physiological process is presented to the patient and/or the therapist as a visual, auditory or tactile signal
- Behavioural modification, defined as the analysis and alteration of the relationship between the patient's symptoms and his/her environment for the treatment of maladaptive voiding patterns [2]

13.1.1.1 Pelvic Floor Muscle Training

The primary conservative treatment of incontinence after radical prostatectomy is pelvic floor muscle training (PFMT) [16].

In contrast to the contemporary PFMT (Kegel exercises), we perform a male-adapted sphincter training (MAST) according to the anatomical research into the external urethral sphincter by Dorschner [6, 7], including behavioural aspects and osteopathic techniques. Our methods are, furthermore, influenced by Feldenkrais' theory [5, 12, 13, 24, 25] (Fig. 13.1.1).

The inpatient rehabilitation programme after radical prostatectomy includes:

- Physiotherapeutic exercises three times a day after initial verbal instructions
- Group physiotherapy for 30 min a day
- Individual single physiotherapy for 30 min three to five times a week

13.1.1.1.1 Verbal Instructions

The patient should be aware of the relevant anatomical structures and the physical functioning of the pelvic floor. The aim of the practical exercises is mobilisation of the spine, proprioceptive recognition and differentiation among the various muscles. A personal strategy is developed by individual adaptation of the exercises.

Male Adapted Sphincter Training (MAST)

instructions about anatomy and of the pelvis and bladder physiology
↓
mobilization of spine, pelvis, hips, bladder
↓
proprioceptive recognition of pelvic muscles
↓
differentiation of antagonistic and agonistic as well as synergistic muscles
↓
special differentiation between urethral and anal sphincter
↓
personalized strategy with individual behavioural training and exercises

Fig. 13.1.1 Male-adapted sphincter training (MAST)

Basic Principles of Continence Exercises

1. None of the exercises should lead to pain or increase existing complaints.
2. Breathing should be calm and steady during the exercises.
3. Inhibition of the sensation of urgency and postponing precautionary voiding.
4. In the case of involuntary urine loss convulsive retaining of urine has to be avoided.

13.1.1.1.2 Mobilisation

The daily continence exercises begin with a mobilisation of spine, bladder, hips and pelvis. This is intended to increase the blood supply to the pelvic organs in order to enable proprioceptive differentiation of agonistic and antagonistic muscles and expansion of the bladder.

Example

The patient lies on his back, eyes closed, relaxed.

The patient should imagine a clockface under his pelvis, 6 o'clock pointing to the head, 12 o'clock to the feet, 3 o'clock to the right and 9 o'clock to the left side.

The pelvis should be moved slightly from 12 to 6, from 1 to 7, from 11 to 5, from 10 to 4, from 2 to 8 and from 3 to 9 o'clock, ten times each.

These movements should be accomplished slowly and without strain. Each movement should be followed by a rest. Sometimes patients experience a sensation of warmth inside the pelvis.

13.1.1.1.3 Proprioceptive Recognition

Imagination of former situations of urgency and recognition of avoiding manoeuvres should help in reorganising the sensorimotor innervation.

13.1.1.1.4 Differentiation of Urethral and Anal Sphincter as Well as Agonistic Muscles

Example 1

Attended by the physiotherapist the patient is instructed to differentiate between the pelvic floor muscles and the external urethral sphincter by placing his hand lightly on the perineum to detect tensing of the pelvic muscles.

Example 2

The patient lies on his back, hands under the buttocks. First he contracts and relaxes the gluteus muscles. Next, he has to contract the urethral sphincter without stretching the gluteus muscles, monitored by his hands.

13.1.1.1.5 Sensorimotor Coordination Exercises

Because of the frequent postoperative loss of sensation in the posterior urethra, the involuntary reflex of sphincter closure has to be facilitated by active exercises, with selective contractions of the urethral sphincter with minimised tension.

The following exercises should be performed ten times each, three times a day:

Example 1

Selective contraction of the sphincter for 1 s and relaxation for 1 s, alternately, like a blinking eyelid.

Example 2

Selective contraction of the sphincter for 3 s and relaxation for 3 s, alternately.

Example 3

Selective contraction of the sphincter for 10 s and relaxation for 10 s, alternately.

13.1.1.1.6 Personalised Strategy with Continuous Behavioural Correction

Basing on the observations of the attending physiotherapist, individual mistakes are corrected continuously. Individual strategies are developed.

Verbal instruction, feedback on contractions and verbal reinforcement of appropriate responses are used to teach contraction of the external urethral sphincter with relaxation of the pelvic muscles. Thus, patients learn to increase intraurethral pressure without increasing abdominal or bladder pressure.

13.1.1.2 Pharmacological Therapy

Concomitant overactive bladder may play a significant role in post-prostatectomy incontinence [17]; therefore, accompanying anticholinergic therapy may be beneficial.

Randomised studies have reported a significant benefit of the additional use of anticholinergic drugs [28]. Additionally, duloxetine may be tried. However, there are currently no evidence-based data supporting the use of duloxetine in this patient group.

13.1.1.3 Biofeedback Therapy

Several techniques of biofeedback therapy are described in the literature but none has been proven effective by randomised controlled studies [8].

A new effective method in the management of urinary incontinence was introduced in 2002 [13]. Of great significance for incontinence seems to be impaired sensitivity of the patient to selective tension of the external urethral sphincter.

Since 1996 we have developed a new method to promote the patient's ability to recognise and exercise the external sphincter via visual perception as a bio-

Videoendoscopic Biofeedback Sphinctertraining

- **visualisati**on of muscle tonus
- **differentiation** of the urethral sphincter tonus
- **perception** of accessory pelvic floor muscles
- continuous **behavioural correction**
- arbitrary, **selective stretching** of the external urethral sphincter
- **Requisition** of hypotone sphincter segments and
- **optimizing** efficacy of tonus

Fig. 13.1.2. Videoendoscopic biofeedback sphincter training

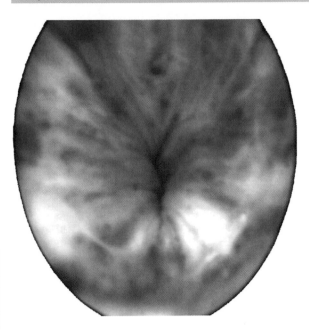

Fig. 13.1.4. External urethral sphincter with tonisation

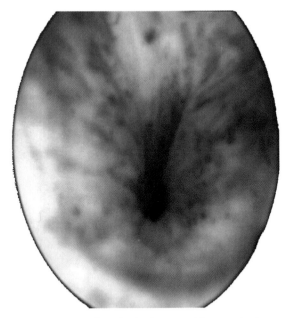

Fig. 13.1.3. External urethral sphincter without tonisation

feedback training method. For this purpose we use a flexible video-endoscope (8 or 15.5 Charrière) to inspect the urethra. Watching the monitor under continuous instruction of the urologist, the patient learns to exercise the external sphincter selectively (Figs. 13.1.2–13.1.4).

In addition, video-endoscopy reveals postoperative complications, e.g. stenosis of the anastomosis, and leads to early therapy (Figs.13.1.5, 13.1.6).

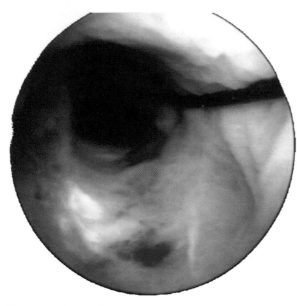

Fig. 13.1.5. Transsphincteric suture

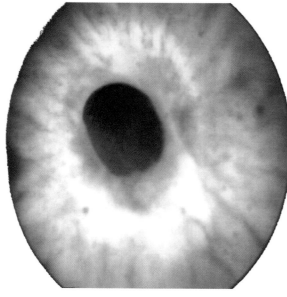

Fig. 13.1.6. Anastomosis stricture

13

13.1.1.4 Electrical Stimulation

Until recently there had only been three studies by one group [36–38] reporting an additional benefit from the use of electrical stimulation.

In 2005 we presented a study that demonstrated a significant advantage for patients using electrical stimulation but only in the case of sufficient compliance [11].

Most former studies denied the benefit of electrical stimulation, but probably insufficient attention was paid to compliance [23, 26, 32, 34].

13.1.2 Algorithms for Conservative Management of Post-Prostatectomy Urinary Incontinence

The algorithms presented in Figs. 13.1.7–13.1.9 have proven successful in the conservative management of post-prostatectomy urinary incontinence.

During the early stages following prostatectomy it is appropriate to institute the described behavioural training, supported by an anticholinergic drug therapy after exclusion of bladder outlet obstruction.

In the first week after removal of the catheter, investigation of leakage can be restricted to the exclusion of infection and an ultrasound check on the completeness of bladder emptying.

If incontinence persists after an initial period of conservative therapy, then urodynamic studies should be undertaken [10].

In addition, video-assisted endoscopic biofeedback sphincter training is efficient.

Deficits in the awareness of voluntary control over the urethral sphincter and increased proprioception of the membranous urethra are detected. The video-biofeedback enables rapid acquisition of visible muscle contraction, achieving strengthening and increasing perseverance.

Patients can be saved from prolonged incorrect and frustrating attempts at pelvic muscle strengthening; instead, they learn adequate active control of the urethral sphincter.

The presented concept of therapy for post-prostatectomy urinary incontinence has proven especially effective in an inpatient rehabilitation programme [25].

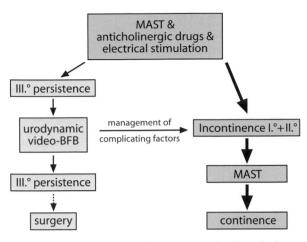

Fig. 13.1.7. Incontinence grade 3. MAST, male-adapted sphincter training; video-BFB, videoendoscopic biofeedback sphincter training

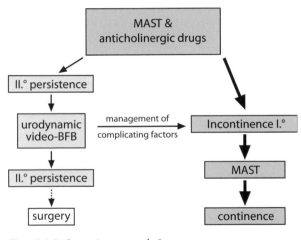

Fig. 13.1.8. Incontinence grade 2

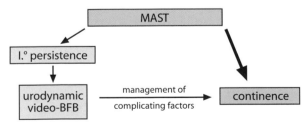

Fig. 13.1.9. Incontinence grade 1

References

1. Abrams P, Cardozo L, Fall M, Griffiths D, Rosier P, Ulmsten U, van Kerrebroeck P, Victor A, Wein A (2002) The standardization of terminology of lower urinary tract function: report from the standardization subcommittee of the International Incontinence Society. Neurourol Urodyn 21:167–178
2. Abrams P, Scientific Committee First ICI (2000) Assessment and treatment of urinary incontinence. Lancet 2000 355:2153–2158
3. Augustin H, Pummer K, Daghofer F, Habermann H, Primus G, Hubmer G (2002) Patient self-reporting questionnaire on urological morbidity and bother after radical prostatectomy. Eur Urol 42:112–117
4. Deliveliotis C, Protogeru V, Alargof E, Varkarakis J (2002) Radical prostatectomy: bladder neck preservation and puboprostatic ligament sparing – effects on continence and positive margins. Urology 60:855–858
5. Dombo O (1999) Rehabilitation der postoperativen Stressinkontinenz beim Mann nach radikaler Prostatovesikulektomie und Zystoprostatektomie. Dissertation, University of Hamburg
6. Dorschner W (1992) Der Streit um den Musculus sphincter urethrae. Histomorphologische Untersuchungen. Akt Urol 23:163–168
7. Dorschner W, Stolzenburg JU (1994) A new theory of micturition and urinary continence based on histomorphological studies. Urol Int 52:185–188
8. Floratos DL, Sonke GS, Rapidou CA et al (2002) Biofeedback versus verbal feedback as learning tools for pelvic muscle exercises in the early management of urinary incontinence after radical prostatectomy. BJU Int 89:714
9. Harris MJ (2003) Radical perineal prostatectomy: cost-efficient, outcome effective, minimally invasive prostate cancer management. Eur Urol 44: 303–308
10. Harrison SCW, Abrams P (1994) Postprostatectomy incontinence. In: Mundy AR, Stephenson TP, Wein AJ (eds) Urodynamics. Churchill Livingstone, New York
11. Hoffmann W, Liedke S, Dombo O, Otto U (2005) Die Elektrostimulation in der Therapie der postoperativen Harninkontinenz nach radikaler Prostatektomie. Urologe A 44:33–40
12. Hoffmann W, Liedke S, Otto U (2002) Das videoendoskopische Biofeedback Sphinktertraining zur Therapie der postoperativen Harninkontinenz nach radikalchirurgischen Operationen. Extracta Urol 3:32–33
13. Hoffmann W, Liedke S, Otto U (2002) Video-endoscopic biofeedback sphincter training for therapy of postoperative urinary incontinence after radical surgery. ICI Paris, Abstract p 53
14. Hofmann T, Gaensheimer S, Buchner A, Rohloff R, Schilling A (1998) An unrandomized prospective comparison of urinary continence, bowel symptoms and the need for further procedures in patients with and with no adjuvant radiation after radical prostatectomy. BJU Int 92:360–364

15. Kielb S, Dunn RL, Rashid MG et al (2002) Assessment of early continence recovery after radical prostatectomy: patient reported symptoms and impairment. J Urol 166:958–961

16. Kondo A, Lin TL, Nordling J, Siroky M, Tammela T (2002) Conservative management in men. In: Incontinence: 2nd International Consultation on Incontinence, Health Publications, Plymbridge

17. Leach GE, Trockman B, Wong A, Hamilton J, Haab F, Zimmern PE (1996) Post-prostatectomy incontinence: urodynamic findings and treatment outcomes. J Urol 155:1256–1259

18. Lepor H, Kaci L (2004) The impact of open radical retropubic prostatectomy on continence and lower urinary tract symptoms: a prospective assessment using validated self-administered outcome instruments. J Urol 171:1216–1219

19. Lowe BA (1996) Comparison of bladder neck preservation to bladder neck resection in maintaining prostatectomy urinary continence. Urology 48(6):889–893

20. Madalinska JW, Essing-Bot ML, Dekoning HJ, Kirkels WJ, van der Maas PJ, Schroder FH (2001) Health-related quality-of-life effects of radical prostatectomy and primary radiotherapy for screen detected or clinically diagnosed localized prostate cancer. J Clin Oncol 19:1619–1628

21. Maffezzini M, Seveso M, Taverna G, Giusti G, Benetti A, Graziotti P (2003) Evaluation of complications and results in a contemporary series of 300 consecutive radial retropubic prostatectomies with the anatomic approach at a single institution. Urology 61:982–986

22. Olsson LE, Salomon L, Nadu A et al (2002) Prospective patient-reported continence after laparoscopic radical prostatectomy. Urology 58:570–572

23. Opsomer RJ, Castille Y, Abi Aad AS, van Cangh PJ (1994) Urinary incontinence after radical prostatectomy: Is professional pelvic floor training necessary? Neurourol Urodyn 13:382–384

24. Otto U, Grosemans P, Hoffmann W, Dombo O (1998) Rehabilitation in der urologischen Onkologie. Urologe B 38 [Suppl 1]:35–40

25. Otto U, Berger D, Krischke NR, Forkel S, Hoffmann W, Petermann F, Klein HO (2002) How effective is the indication-specific inpatient-rehabilitation of cancer patients after radical prostatectomy? J Cancer Res Clin Oncol 126 [Suppl]:109

26. Pannek J, König JE (2005) Clinical usefulness of pelvic floor reeducation for men undergoing radical prostatectomy. Urol Int 74:38–43

27. Rassweiler J, Seemann O, Schulze M, Teber D, Hatzinger M, Frede T (2003) Laparoscopic versus open radical prostatectomy: a comparative study at a single institution. J Urol 169: 1689–1693

28. Rudy D, Clein K, Goldberg K, Harris R (2004) A multicenter randomized, placebo-controlled trial of trospium chloride in overactive bladder patients. Neurourol Urodyn 23:600–601 (abstr. 144)

29. Ruiz-Deya G, Davis R, Srivastav SK, A MW, Thomas R (2001) Outpatient radical prostatectomy: impact of standard perineal approach on patient outcome. J Urol 166:581–586

30. Sebesta M, Cespedes RD, Luhman E, Optenberg S, Thompson IM (2002) Questionnaire-based outcomes of urinary incontinence and satisfaction rates after radical prostatectomy in an national study population. Urology 60:1055–1058

31. Stolzenburg JU, Waldkirch E, Do M, Rabenalt R, Do M, Ho KMT, Dorschner W, Horn L, Jonas U, Truss MC (2005) Endoscopic extraperitoneal radical prostatectomy (EE-RPE) – oncological and functional results after 700 procedures, J Urol 174:1271–1275

32. Temml C, Haidinger C, Schmidbauer J et al. (2000) Urinary incontinence in both sexes: prevalence rates and impact on quality of life and sexual life. Neurourol Urodyn 19:259

33. Van Kampen M, De Weerdt W, Van Poppel H, De Ridder D, Feys H, Baert L (2000) Effect of pelvic floor re-education on duration and degree of incontinence after radical prostatectomy: a randomised controlled trial. Lancet 355:98–102

34. Wei, JT, Dunn RL, Marcovich R, Montie JE, Sanda MG (2000) Prospective assessment of patient-reported urinary continence after radical prostatectomy. J Urol 164:744–748

35. Wille S, Sobottka A, Heidenreich A, Hofmann R (2003) Pelvic floor exercises, electrical stimulation and biofeedback after radical prostatectomy: results of a prospective randomized trial. J Urol 170 (2 Pt 1):490–493

36. Yamanishi T, Yasuda K (1998) Electrical stimulation for stress incontinence. Int Urogynecol J Pelvic Floor Dysfunct 9:281

37. Yamanishi T, Yasuda K, Sakakibara R et al (2000) Randomised double-blind study of electrical stimulation for urinary incontinence due to detrusor overactivity. Urology 55:353

38. Yasuda K, Yamanishi T (1999) Critical evaluation of electrostimulation for management of female urinary incontinence. Curr Opin Obstet Gynecol 11:503

13

Rehabilitation of Erectile Function After Radical Prostatectomy

13.2

Klaus-Peter Jünemann

Radical prostatectomy is the standard procedure for locally confined prostate cancer with respect to progression-free long-term survival, PSA progression-free survival and total survival [14]. Clinical long-term follow-up data demonstrate satisfactory cancer control with concurrent acceptable quality of life [1, 14]. With his studies on the anatomy of the prostate and the neurovascular bundles which run in close proximity of the prostate toward the penile corpora cavernosa, Walsh [2], in the mid-1980's, established the "anatomical radical prostatectomy" and thus paved the way for the currently established surgical technique of radical prostatectomy. By means of this surgical procedure and the subsequent multiple modifications, it was possible to reduce the therapy-related erectile dysfunction rates from nearly 100% to 30%–60% in specialized centres (Table 13.2.1). If a nerve-sparing procedure was performed, these results can

be expected with a delay of several weeks to 25 months post surgery [3–6].

Meticulous bilateral preservation of the neurovascular bundle, which requires anatomical and physiological knowledge of the erectile mechanism, as well as extensive experience and fine skill on the part of the surgeon, will ensure that around 56% of preoperatively potent patients will be able to achieve full rigid erections, sufficient for sexual intercourse, without additional help. When adding to this figure those patients who respond to therapy with phosphodiesterase-5 (PDE-5) inhibitors, the rate of postoperative erectile capability is as high as 90% [7].

One should be aware that the postoperative period required for recovery of a full rigid erection plays a significant role. In a highly selective group of patients (n=64) with locally confined prostate cancer (98.5% pT1 or pT2, 87% Gleason score≤6), 89% of whom un-

Table 13.2.1. Published erection rates after nerve-sparing radical prostatectomy. One surgeon's experience with a minimum follow-up of 12 months in all series

Author	Spontaneous erections	+ PDE-5 I
Catalona (1999)	68% bilateral	Ø
	47% unilateral	Ø
Stanford (2000)	–	44% bilateral
	–	42% unilateral
	–	35% non-nerve-sparing
Huland (2003)	37–69% bilateral	84–97%
	18–37% unilateral	64–76%
Lepor (2005)	<50 years	78%
	50 years	63%
Menon (2006)	71%	96%
Jünemann (2007)	47% 1 year PDE-5 I*	86%
	28% 1 year without PDE-5 I*	66%

* PDE-5 I at night, 25 mg sildenafil daily at night

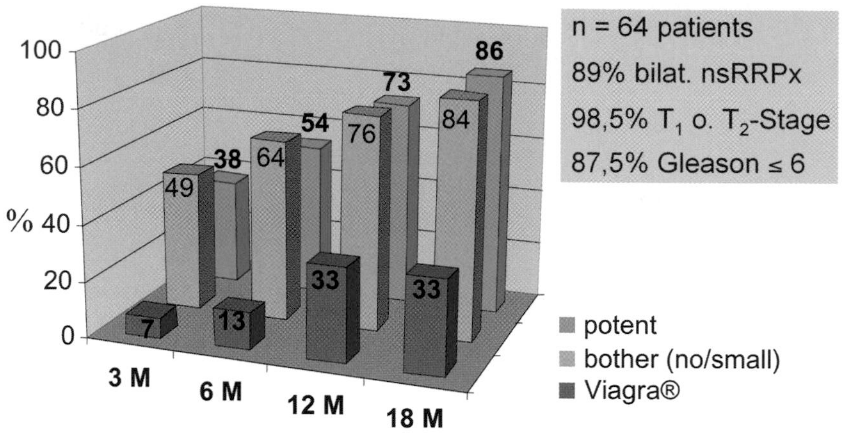
n = 64 patients
89% bilat. nsRRPx
98,5% T_1 o. T_2-Stage
87,5% Gleason ≤ 6
100
80
60
% 40
20
0
3 M
6 M
12 M
18 M
49
7
38
64
13
54
76
33
73
84
33
86
potent
bother (no/small)
Viagra®

Fig. 13.2.1. Patient-reported potency rates after nerve-sparing radical prostatectomy over 18 months' follow-up according to Walsh et al. [3]

Table 13.2.2. Factors influencing successful use of sildenafil citrate after nerve-sparing and non-nerve-sparing radical prostatectomy (n=147 patients).

Factors	Success rates (sildenafil response)
Nerve-sparing	71%
Non-nerve-sparing	14%
Preoperative IIEF 5: <15/≥16	27%/68%
Age (years): <60/60–65/>65	76%/57%/43%
Time after operation (months): 3–6/6–12/12–18/>18	0%/57%/63%/91%

Success is defined as positive and sufficient erectile response to sildenafil citrate [15]

derwent bilateral nerve-sparing radical prostatectomy, Walsh et al. [3] has been able to show that within 18 months after the intervention, the rate of erectile response sufficient for sexual intercourse rose from 38% at 3 months to 86% at 18 months follow-up (Fig. 13.2.1). A remarkable aspect in this prospective study is the fact that 33% of the 86% responders routinely used sildenafil (Viagra®) to achieve sufficient erectile quality and rigidity. As many as 84% of the men investigated during follow-up did not report any impairment in their sexuality.

For a successful erectile outcome, the decisive factors, according to Raina et al. [15], are (Table 13.2.2):

1. Nerve-sparing surgical technique
2. Preoperative erectile status
3. Patient age

Raina and co-workers [15] demonstrate that a response to sildenafil sufficient for recovery of erectile capability is chiefly dependent on the time that has elapsed since the surgical intervention: 57% at 6–12 months, 63% at 12–18 months, and 91% at 18 months and longer.

Particularly the delayed recovery of erectile capability, with or without the use of a PDE-5 inhibitor, raises the question of the pathophysiological causes and mechanisms behind postoperative erectile dysfunction.

13.2.1 Pathophysiology of Erectile Dysfunction After Nerve-sparing Radical Prostatectomy

The pathophysiological mechanism of the surgically induced erectile dysfunction after radical prostatectomy cannot be explained here in detail; however, the basic principles of erectile induction as well as erectile maintenance, and their impairment by surgical intervention will be outlined in brief. For further informa-

Fig. 13.2.2. Pathophysiology and erectile rehabilitation after radical prostatectomy (from [12] with permission of the authors)

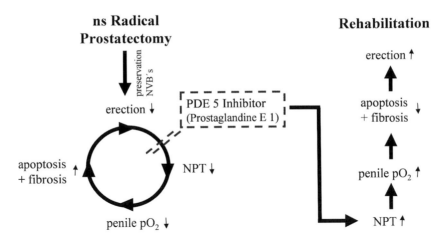

tion we refer the reader to van der Horst et al. [12] and McCullough [13].

The most intriguing question in connection with the radical prostatectomy procedure is what happens with the neurovascular bundle and subsequently the erectile tissue:

1. The surgery induces a parasympathetic neuropraxia or denervation, leading to a loss of neuronal nitric oxide synthase (NOS).
2. The penis has an unbalanced sympathetic tone, resulting in a state of constant muscle contraction.
3. Oxygenation of the corpora cavernosa, particularly during nocturnal penile tumescence (REM sleep), is reduced or completely abolished, resulting in intracorporal fibrosis and subsequent apoptosis of the smooth musculature, eventually leading to penile atrophy.
4. Clinical studies have documented that veno-occlusive dysfunction is present in 40% of patients with erectile dysfunction after radical prostatectomy (diminished intracavernosal smooth muscular relaxation).

Reduction in penile length, in particular, which is usually noticed by the affected patients between 6 and 12 months after surgery, presents a clinical proof of these pathophysiological effects. Penile shortening is the result of hypoxically induced atrophy of the corpora cavernosa. This is contradictory to what was commonly believed previously, namely that the shortening of the penile shaft was related to surgical anastomosis between the urethral stump and the bladder neck after removal of the prostate, leading to intrapelvic tension of the urethra with subsequent shortening of the entire penis. This seemingly logical and simple explanation is obviously wrong; the reduction in penile length is in fact related to the hypoxia-induced fibrosis within the corpora cavernosa and thus induction of apoptosis of the smooth musculature within the erectile tissue [8–13] (Fig. 13.2.2).

In the same context it seems that the oxygen that enables nocturnal penile erections plays a significant role in preserving the smooth muscle content of the corpora cavernosa: with a non-nerve-sparing procedure, or if the nerve fibres stretching towards the penis suffer substantial impairment or destruction, the smooth muscles are no longer oxygenated at night.

Although the hypothesis of the protective influence of sufficient oxygenation of the corpora cavernosa has not yet been proven, a significant amount of evidence, both clinical and experimental, indicates that preservation of the nocturnal erectile capability is the main factor for guaranteeing the survival of the smooth musculature of the erectile tissue [12, 13].

It is without doubt that the intensity of nocturnal erectile episodes after intrapelvic surgery is reduced, and they may also be less frequent. This raises the question of the relevance of nocturnal smooth muscle oxygenation for protection of the erectile mechanism.

Wayman and co-workers [16] demonstrated, in a preclinical experimental model, that the reduction of the arterial inflow to the penis impairs erectile capa-

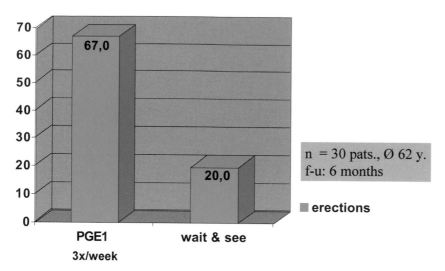

Fig. 13.2.3. Recovery of spontaneous erectile function after nerve-sparing radical prostatectomy with or without intracavernous injections of PGE1 (n=30 patients, mean age 62 years, follow-up 6 months). According to Montorsi et al. [18]

bility and/or significantly reduces penile rigidity. The molecular-biological background for this pathophysiological mechanism is a reduction in endothelial NOS (eNOS) that is directly related to sufficient oxygenation of the vascular and smooth muscular structures to and within the penis [20]. Wayman and co-workers were able to decode the pathomechanism of erectile dysfunction with impaired oxygenation: a remarkable finding in their experimental studies was that – while the arterial inflow was equally reduced – the erectile quality, particularly the rigidity, recovered completely with the addition a PDE-5 inhibitor, in this case sildenafil, due to the improved oxygenation of the corpora cavernosa [17]. The latter observation permits the hypothesis that recovery of erectile function after radical prostatectomy or any other intrapelvic surgery may be achieved by utilizing or adding a vasoactive drug or even a PDE-5 inhibitor.

13.2.2 Rehabilitation Concept After Radical Prostatectomy

The question of whether preoperatively existing erectile capability can be preserved or recovered postoperatively is often crucial for the patient as well as for the clinician, who usually decides which form of treatment (surgery or brachytherapy) is to be applied. The potential of rehabilitation of the smooth musculature through stimulation with a vasoactive agent was first shown by Montorsi and co-workers [18]. In a prospective study on 30 patients with a mean age of 62 years and 6 months follow-up, who had undergone nerve-sparing radical prostatectomy, the patients were randomized in two groups of 15 patients each. Group I received corpus cavernosum injection therapy with prostaglandin E1 (PGE1) 3×/week, while group II did not receive any additional injection therapy. After 6 months, 67% of the patients who underwent PGE1 stimulation of the cavernous tissue reported full rigid erection sufficient for sexual intercourse, against 20% of those in the "wait-and-see" group without vasoactive stimulation (Fig. 13.2.3). On the basis of their preliminary results, the authors concluded that continuous and regular stimulation of the smooth musculature of the corpus cavernosum proved sufficient for recovery of erectile function.

Not every patient who undergoes nerve-sparing radical prostatectomy is suitable for auto-injection PGE1 therapy after the surgical procedure. Therefore the question arises of whether regular intake of a PDE-5 inhibitor would lead to results as promising as those described by Montorsi with PGE1 injections 3×/week.

In order to understand the principle of PDE-5-inhibitor-induced smooth muscle rehabilitation of the corpora cavernosa, a second study by Montorsi and colleagues [19] needs to be discussed. Patients with erectile dysfunction without any previous intrapelvic surgery or prostate cancer underwent measurement of nocturnal penile tumescence and rigidity (NPTR) before commencing a routine of sildenafil intake every night.

Fig. 13.2.4. Nocturnal penile tumescence and rigidity (NPTR) in patients with impaired erectile function (pathological NPTR) and after 100 mg sildenafil on two consecutive nights in an impotent patient, 50 years old, a heavy smoker, with hypertension and hyperlipidaemia. The second recording demonstrates a significant improvement in frequency of erectile episodes and rigidity of the erectile response at night [19]

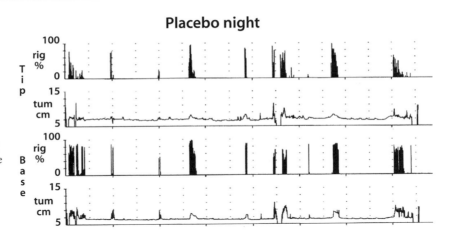

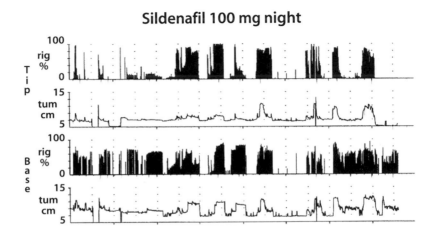

The first NPTR recording, before the administration of sildenafil, demonstrated impaired, sometimes highly pathological, nocturnal penile tumescence, correlating well with the patients' complaint of significant erectile dysfunction. The patients then received 100 mg sildenafil for two consecutive nights [19]. During each night the NPTR measurements were repeated. As shown in Fig. 13.2.4, the recording after two consecutive nights of administration of sildenafil in the same patients demonstrates a significant increase in the frequency and duration of the erectile episodes and in the degree of rigidity. This important paper was the first to describe the improvement of nocturnal penile capability in impotent men by regular intake of a PDE-5 inhibitor.

Based on these results, the question arises of whether an improved erectile status at night would be helpful in the recovery and rehabilitation of erectile quality in patients after nerve-sparing radical prostatectomy. A first indication that this hypothesis could be valid was provided by a study by Sommer and co-workers [21], who performed a prospective study on 112 mildly to moderately impotent men, all of whom were responders to PDE-5 inhibitors. The patients were randomized into three different groups. Group I received 50 mg sildenafil daily, group II used 50 mg or 100 mg sildenafil as required only for intercourse, and group III received no further treatment. The therapy was continued for 1 year and then stopped. One month later, the patients were interviewed concerning their spontaneous erectile capability without additional PDE-5 inhibitor intake. The results were astonishing: in group III, with no further treatment, 5.6% of patients reported spontaneous erections; in group II, who had used 50–100 mg sildenafil on demand, the rate was 8.2%; and in group I, who had received 50 mg sildenafil daily, 60.4% of patients reported spontaneous erections without the application of sildenafil or any other PDE-5 inhibitor. Additionally, duplex sonography of the penis demonstrated significantly improved arterial inflow into the smooth musculature in group I.

13.2.3 The Kiel Concept

When integrating the basic signs and clinical results to derive a rehabilitation concept for the corpora cavernosa after nerve-sparing radical prostatectomy, it seems logical to follow the principle of prophylactic smooth muscle preservation [12, 13] (Fig. 13.2.2), i.e. regular administration of low dose PDE-5 inhibitor in order to improve the oxygenation of the smooth musculature of the penis, thus reducing or preventing fibrosis within the corporeal smooth musculature, which will in turn prevent apoptosis and restore erectile capability

Based on these considerations, a prospective study was conducted by the present authors' work group. Initially, nocturnal penile tumescence, rigidity and erection quality were measured after nerve-sparing radical prostatectomy [22].

In 43 patients who underwent radical prostatectomy with uni- or bilateral preservation of the neurovascular bundle, an NPTR measurement was performed the night following the removal of the catheter in the clinic. Evaluation of the recording revealed that 41 out of 43 patients (95%) showed sufficiently rigid erections as early as 7–14 days after the surgical procedure. An NPTR erection was considered "normal" if 70% of the maximum erectile rigidity was achieved over a duration of at least 10 min. In order to validate the technique, five patients operated on with a non-nerve-sparing procedure underwent the same NPTR recording at night and showed no erections at all. By means of such post-surgical measurements it is possible to prove, or at least to evaluate, the success of the nerve-sparing procedure on the basis of more or less objective criteria.

In a second step, the 41 patients who had shown sufficient nocturnal erections (1–5) were divided into two subgroups: the patients in group I (n=23) received 25 mg sildenafil every night and were compared to a control group without additional medication (group

II; n=18). In all patients the preoperative erectile status had been evaluated by means of the IIEF-5 score. All patients in both groups reached a comparable IIEF score of slightly above 20 (fully potent). The patients were followed up at 6, 12, 24, 36 and 52 weeks after surgery and filled out the IIEF questionnaire each time [23].

While within the first 6 months no or only insignificant differences were found between the two groups (Fig. 13.2.5), significant differences emerged at 36 weeks and after 1 year, manifesting themselves as higher IIEF scores in the sildenafil group. The patients who received 25 mg sildenafil at night showed better erectile capability than those who had received no additional treatment.

The questionnaire further revealed that after 1 year, 86% of the patients who took 25 mg sildenafil every night reported spontaneous erections sufficient for intercourse (Table 13.2.1). Around 60% of these patients did not require any additional PDE-5 inhibitors/sildenafil, while almost 40% took 25 mg or even 50 mg Viagra® on demand to further improve erectile quality. In the control group, 35% of the patients reported full rigid erections without additional sildenafil and 65% made use of a PDE-5 inhibitor. Overall, 66% of the patients in the control group reported rigid erections with or without the use of sildenafil (Table 13.2.1).

This study is still under way but demonstrates even at this stage that regular low-dose administration of sildenafil improves the erectile capability, and, much more significantly, restores the patient's capacity for a rewarding sex life.

On the basis of these study results, we have drawn up the "Kiel concept", which relies on the described data of low-dose administration of sildenafil or, probably, other PDE-5 inhibitors [23] (Fig. 13.2.6). This concept provides for patients who report spontaneous nocturnal erections to receive 25 mg Viagra® daily after discharge from the clinic. Smooth muscle stimulation of the corpora cavernosa with sildenafil is performed over a period of at least 3 months, with a first so-called „Viagra® test" after 8 weeks to test the spontaneous erectile capability after the training programme. In order to do so, the patient has a minimum of four attempts with 50–100 mg Viagra® under sexual stimulation from the partner. Depending on the erectile results, the low-dose PDE-5 inhibitor smooth muscle stimulation should be continued until spontaneous erections sufficient for sexual intercourse can be achieved, even if only with intake of additional

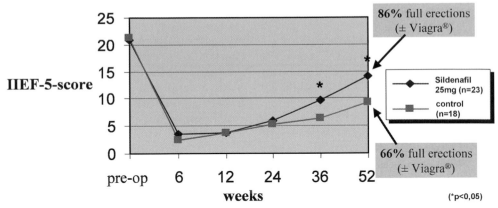

Fig. 13.2.5. Recovery of erectile function after nerve-sparing radical prostatectomy with and without low-dose sildenafil daily for 1 year. At 36 weeks after surgery the IIEF-5 scores are significantly different, and at 52 weeks the sildenafil group shows erections sufficient for intercourse in 86% of patients, compared with 66% in the control group (no sildenafil daily) (from [23] with permission of the authors)

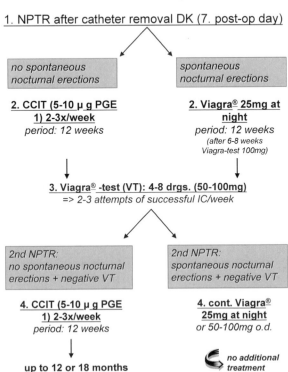

Fig. 13.2.6. The Kiel concept. Since 95% of all our patients that underwent uni- or bilateral nerve-sparing radical prostatectomy demonstrated sufficient erections during the first night after catheter removal, the low-dose sildenafil therapy could be initiated right away [24]

PDE-5 inhibitor. This rehabilitation scheme should be continued for up to 12 or even 18 months, according to Walsh's findings from the year 2000 [3], to exploit the maximum rehabilitative potential of chronic PDE-5 inhibitor stimulation of the penile smooth musculature. At regular intervals of 6, subsequently 9 and 12 months, further attempts of sexual intercourse are to be performed with a high-dose intake of 50 mg or 100 mg Viagra® or a similar PDE-5 inhibitor to test the erectile status.

If the patient shows no nocturnal erections, or if the NPTR recording after 3 months shows no response to a PDE-5 inhibitor stimulation, even under high-dose administration of Viagra® (Viagra® test), it is advisable to switch to administration of PGE1 2–3×/week for the next 3 months. At the end of this time the erectile results are re-evaluated with another Viagra® test [24] (Fig. 13.2.6).

Although the Kiel concept has proved successful in the restoration of erectile capability after nerve-sparing radical prostatectomy, the question remains open whether PDE-5 inhibitors such as tadalafil and vardenafil have the same potential as sildenafil to restore the smooth musculature of the corporal tissue after the surgical procedure.

13.2.4 Conclusion

It can be concluded that sufficient oxygenation of the smooth musculature of the corpora cavernosa after nerve-sparing radical prostatectomy is relevant for preservation of erectile function. Sildenafil, and probably other PDE-5 inhibitors, improve smooth muscle oxygenation of the corpora cavernosa, thus preventing the induction of smooth muscular fibrosis and consecutive apoptosis. By preserving the smooth musculature erectile tissue, full restoration of erectile capability after intrapelvic surgery, in particular nerve-sparing radical prostatectomy, can be achieved.

As our own study results demonstrate, daily or nightly low-dose administration of sildenafil (Viagra®), and probably of other PDE-5 inhibitors, as described by the Kiel concept, is helpful in obtaining rapid partial or complete restoration of the erectile function after surgical intervention. In the long term, a benefit for patients who underwent chronic stimula-

tion with sildenafil could be demonstrated by comparison with a control group.

The question remains open, however, of whether nightly/daily application of a low-dose PDE-5 inhibitor is necessary or whether intake every second day would be sufficient. Furthermore, it needs to be mentioned that the most important prerequisite for a rehabilitation of the smooth musculature of the erectile tissue, according to the Kiel concept, lies in the quality of the nerve-sparing functional surgical procedure and the skill of the surgeon who performs it.

References

1. Han M, Partin AW, Pound CR, Epstein JI, Walsh PC (2001) Long term biochemical disease-free and cancer-specific survival following anatomic radical retropubic prostatectomy.The 15-year Johns Hopkins experience.Urol Clin North Am 28:555–565
2. Walsh PC (1988) Preservation of sexual function in the surgical treatment of prostatic cancer-an anatomic surgical approach. In: Devita VT, Hellman S, Rosenberg S (eds) Important advances in oncology. Lippincott, Philadelphia, pp 161–170
3. Walsh PC, Marschke P, Ricker D, Burnett AL (2000) Patient-reported urinary continence and sexual function after anatomic radical prostatectomy. Urology 55:58–61
4. Walsh PC, Partin AW, Epstein JI (1994) Cancer control and quality of life following anatomical radical retropubic prostatectomy: results at 10 years. J Urol 152:1831–1836
5. Catalona WJ, Carvalhal GF, Mager DE, Smith DS (1999) Potency, continence and complication rates in 1,870 consecutive radical retropubic prostatectomies. J Urol 162:433–438
6. Rabbani F, Stapleton AM, Kattan MW, Wheeler TM, Scardino PT (2000) Factors predicting recovery of erections after radical prostatectomy. J Urol 164:1929–1934
7. Michl U, Graefen M, Noldus J, Eggert T, Huland H (2003) Functional results of various surgical techniques for radical prostatectomy. Urologe A 42:1196–1202
8. Wespes E (2000) Erectile dysfunction in the ageing man. Curr Opin Urol 10:625–628
9. Liu X, Lin CS, Graziottin T, Resplande J, Lue TF (2001) Vascular endothelial growth factor promotes proliferation and migration of cavernous smooth muscle cells. J Urol 166:354–360
10. Moreland RB (1998) Is there a role of hypoxemia in penile fibrosis: a viewpoint presented to the Society for the Study of Impotence. Int J Impot Res 10:113–120
11. User HM, Hairston JH, Zelner DJ, Mc Kenna KE, McVary KT (2003) Penile weight and cell subtype specific changes in a post radical prostatectomy model of erectile dysfunction. J Urol 169:1175–1179

12. van der Horst C, Martinez-Portillo FJ, Jünemann KP (2005) Pathophysiologie und Rehabilitation der erectilen Dysfunktion nach nerverhaltender radikaler Prostatektomie. Urologe A 44:667–673

13. McCullough AR (2001) Prevention and management of erectile dysfunction following radical prostatectomy. Urol Clin North Am 28:613–627

14. Porter CR, Kodama K, Gibbons RP, Correa R Jr, Chun FK, Perrotte P, Karakiewicz PI (2006) 25-year prostate cancer control and survival outcomes: a 40 year radical prostatectomy single institution series. J Urol 176:569–74

15. Raina R, Nelson DR, Agrawal A, Lakin MM, Klein EA, Zippe CD (2002) Long term efficacy of sildenafil citrate following radical prostatectomy: 3-year follow-up. J Urol 167 [Suppl 4]:279

16. Wayman C, Hornby S, Burden A, Casey J (2005) Sildenafil increases erection hardness by potentiating pudendal artery blood flow in the anaesthetised dog. Proceedings, 8th Congress of ESSM, Copenhagen, Denmark

17. Wayman C, Hornby S, Burden A, Casey J (2005) Sildenafil increases erection hardness by improved penile oxygenation in the anaesthetised dog. Proceedings, 8th Congress of ESSM, Copenhagen, Denmark

18. Montorsi F, Guazzoni G, Strambi LF, Da Pozzo LF, Nava, L, Barbieri L, Rigatti P, Pizzini G, Miani A (1997) Recovery of spontaneous erectile function after nerve-sparing radical retropubic prostatectomy with and without early intracavernous injections of alprostadil: results of a prospective, randomized trial. J Urol 158:1408–1410

19. Montorsi F, Maga T, Strambi LF, Salonia A, Barbieri L, Scattoni V, Guazzoni G, Losa A, Rigatti P, Pizzini G (2000) Sildenafil taken at bedtime significantly increases nocturnal erections: results of a placebo-controlled study. Urology 56:906–911

20. Hurt KJ, Musicki B, Palese MA, Crone JK, Becker RE, Moriarity JL, Snyder SH, Burnett AL (2002) Akt-dependent phosphorylation of endothelial nitric oxide synthase mediates penile erection. Proc Natl Acad Sci 99:4061–4066

21. Sommer F, Klotz T, Engelmann U (2007) Improved spontaneous erectile function in men with mild-to-moderate arteriogenic erectile dysfunction treated with a nightly dose of sildenafil for one year: a randomized trial. Asian J Androl 9:134–141

22. Bannowsky A, Schulze H, van der Horst C, Seif C, Braun PM, Jünemann KP (2006) Nocturnal tumescence: a parameter for postoperative erectile integrity after nerve sparing radical prostatectomy. J Urol 175:2214–2217

23. Bannowsky A, Schulze, H, van der Horst C, Hautmann, S, Braun PM, Jünemann KP (2007) Recovery of erectile function after nerve-sparing radical prostatectomy – improvement with nightly low dose sildenafil. J Urol (submitted)

24. Bannowsky A, Schulze H, van der Horst C, Stübinger, JH, Portillo FJ, Jünemann KP (2005) Erectile function after nerve-sparing radical prostatectomy. Nocturnal early erection as a parameter of postoperative organic erectile integrity. Urologe A 44:521–526